The Urinal Of Physick

Robert Recorde

The Urinal of Physick

A Facsimile of the
First Edition
Imprinted at London by
Reynolde Wolfe
1547

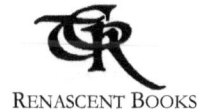

Renascent Books

PUBLICATION HISTORY

THE URINAL OF PHYSICK
First imprinted by Reynolde Wolfe in 1547

Subsequent Editions
Imprinted by Reynolde Wolfe
1548, 1558, 1559
Imprinted by Reginalde Wolf
1567, 1574, 1582
Imprinted by Thomas Dawson
1599
Printed by Gartrude Dawson
1651
Printed by G. D.
1665
Printed by Peter Parker
as
THE JUDGMENT OF URINES
1679

Hardback facsimile edition published by
TGR Renascent Books
27 Springdale Court
Mickleover, Derby DE3 9SW
United Kingdom
2011

Paperback edition first published 2012

All rights reserved. No part of this publication may be reproduced, stored in a retrieval system, or transmitted, in any form or by any means, without the prior permission in writing of the publisher, or as expressly permitted by law.

© Thomas Gordon Roberts 2011

ISBN 978-1-4793231-2-8
www.renascentbooks.co.uk

Printed and bound by
CreateSpace, Charleston, South Carolina, U.S.A.

for
JOAN

INTRODUCTION

This book is a facsimile of Robert Recorde's *The Urinal of Physick*, originally printed in London by Reynolde Wolfe in 1547. The work is an early urological treatise, concerned with the practice of making diagnoses by inspecting the patient's urine. Robert Recorde was a physician at the courts of Henry VIII, Edward VI and Mary I; he was also a very learned scholar and mathematician, a teacher of outstanding ability and a skilful textbook writer. He wrote a progression of justly famed mathematical textbooks with the following titles: *The Grounde of Artes, The Pathway to Knowledge, The Gate of Knowledge, The Castle of Knowledge, The Treasure of Knowledge* and *The Whetstone of Witte*. Of these six, *The Gate* and *The Treasure* are no longer extant and *The Castle* deals with Ptolemaic astronomy rather than the study of mathematics *per se*. Recorde was also learned in medicine and law and was familiar with Greek and medieval texts as well as contemporary developments. He was an able Greek scholar who insisted that a knowledge of that language was important for an accurate understanding of sources; he was a historian interested in the antiquities of Britain, a collector of manuscripts and probably one of the first students of the Anglo-Saxon language. In short, he was a consummate Renaissance man. Despite the foregoing, Recorde had no international reputation, probably because all of his works were in English (rather than Latin, the scholarly language of his day) and were on an elementary level. In England however, his mathematical books remained the standard texts throughout the Elizabethan period. A generation of English navigators and scientific practitioners, especially non-university men, stated that Recorde's books had

Introduction

been their first tutors in the mathematical sciences.

Recorde graduated B.A. from Oxford in 1531 and was subsequently elected a fellow of All Souls College in the same year. All Souls was a chantry and graduate foundation for the study and training of clerks in theology, civil and cannon law and medicine. At some time he left Oxford for Cambridge and there received an M.D. degree in 1545. According to Cambridge records he had been licensed in medicine at Oxford some twelve years earlier, and the Cambridge M.D. usually went with an Oxford license. His only extant medical treatise, *The Urinal of Physick*, dedicated to the Company of Surgeons, is signed 'At my house in London. 8 Novemb. 1547.', so he was probably practising medicine there at this time. In the dedication he promises a work on anatomy, which if actually written has not survived. At the end of the book he gives a summary (A Universal Table) which he concludes by saying 'More largely have I written thereof in a book of the same title, but in the Latin tongue, as more meet for learned ears, & for them that need more precise judgement'. This work, if published, has also not survived. *The Urinal* is a traditional text on the judgement of urines, full of sensible nursing practice in accordance with the mores of the time. However, it is less modern than his mathematical texts and much less critical of authority. Throughout the book, Record quotes the opinions and teaching of classical authors such as Hippocrates, Galen, Avicenna and many others, without criticism or amendment. This is in stark contrast to his mathematical works, in all of which he urges his readers to use their own reason and observation as a guide to truth, before uncritically accepting the teachings of ancient authorities. Nevertheless, *The Urinal* was a successful book. It remained in print for over 130 years and after the publication of the first edition was

Introduction

reprinted no less than ten times. The following notes are provided as a guide to reading and understanding this fascinating medical textbook.

PAGINATION

Pages are not numbered individually as in modern practice; rather each leaf only is numbered on the right-hand side. However, the original compositors have confused the leaf numbering. Ordering starts with the preface (the leaves of the dedication are not numbered) and proceeds to 31, whereupon the next leaf is numbered 34. Numbering then continues correctly from 33 to 36, followed incorrectly by 39 and 29, correctly by 39 to 56 and then 37 instead of 57. Thereafter the numbering is correct to the finish of the text, although the table at the end of the book is not numbered. In summary, the book has two leaves numbered 29, two numbered 34, two numbered 37 and two numbered 39. Contrariwise, there are no leaves numbered 32, 37, 38 and 57. However, for the benefit of modern day readers who expect consistent pagination, modern page numbering is applied over a line drawn above Recorde's text.

SPELLINGS AND PUNCTUATION

Dictionaries and standard spellings did not exist when *The Urinal of Physick* was first printed, and many words are not even spelt phonetically. Therefore many spellings in the book appear peculiar to the modern reader, but a little practice at reading Early Modern English soon renders the text intelligible. Many familiar words look strange simply because, unlike modern spellings, they end with the silent letter e and the last consonant might or might not be doubled, hence *mane* or *manne* (man), and *rune* or *runne* (run). The letter y is often used in place of i, for example *fyrste* (first) or *tryckle* (trickle). Early printing conventions were to use the terminal letter s at the end

Introduction

of words, as today, but the long form everywhere else, for example *poſſeſs* (possess). The letters u and v were not considered to be two distinct letters, but different forms of the same letter. Typographically, v was often used at the start of words and u elsewhere, hence *vrine* (urine) and *vnloued* (unloved). But conversely, the letter v was often used where today we would expect the letter u, as in, for example, *thervnto* (thereunto). Neither were the letters i and j considered distinct, so that the word judicial would be spelt *ivdicial*. In short, and for example, expect to read modern spellings such as some, division and judge, as *ſomme, diuiſion* and *ivdge*.

Punctuation appears eccentric to modern eyes – for example, commas are sometimes present when (by modern standards) their use is not required. Conversely they are often missing where present-day usage would insert them. Often a forward slash / is used in place of a comma, semi-colon or a full stop. Full stops and the colon are used arbitrarily and interchangeably, and the ends of sentences are sometimes not terminated by any punctuation at all. The first word of a following sentence might or might not be capitalised. Another peculiarity in the text is the use of the letter y where today we would use an apostrophe, for example *mannys* (man's).

CONTRACTIONS

Throughout the book, the words 'the' and 'that' are contracted to y^e and y^t respectively, with the small letters e and t placed directly above the y. Of course, these words should be read with their full pronunciation – 'the' and 'that'. The word 'with' is often contracted to w^t, again with the t in smaller point directly above the w. Occasionally this contraction is encountered in combination, e.g. w^t + out (w^tout) for 'without', as on line 23, leaf 31r. A distinctive symbol p is sometimes used by the compositors of *The Urinal* to represent 'per' or 'pro',

Introduction

so that 'perceive' for example, might appear spelt phonetically in full as 'perceyue', or as on line 23, leaf 4v, contracted to ꝑceyue. Again, as on line 19, leaf 23v the word 'perfyte' (perfect) is contracted to ꝑfyte, and on line 22, leaf 15r the word 'proper' is contracted to ꝑper. Likewise, the symbol ᵥ is used to represent 'ver', as on line 20, leaf 68v, where the word 'vertues' is contracted to ᵥtues, or line 22, leaf 71r where 'universall' (universal) is contracted to uniᵥsall. Another peculiarity is the spelling of Latin names, where 'us' is represented by an apostrophe. An example is found on line 3, leaf 2v of the preface, where the name Cornelius is contracted to Corneli'.

DIACRITICAL MARKS

Diacritical marks have been used to abbreviate printed words ever since Gutenberg, and early English printers adopted the same conventions that Gutenberg did for Latin texts (which he copied, in turn, from the handwritten texts of medieval scribes). Diacritical marks are used on most pages of *The Urinal of Physick* to indicate the omission of the consonant m or n where this follows a vowel. The missing letter is indicated by placing a mark over the vowel. Instances are *understād* (understand), *mē* (men), *touchīg* (touching), *physiciō* (physicion - physician), and *substaūce* (substaunce – substance). Many words are shortened with more than one diacritical mark, for example *cōtinuīg* (continuing). Words abbreviated with diacritical marks should also be read, of course, with their full pronunciation.

TYPOGRAPHICAL FEATURES

All the contractions and abbreviations found in the pages of *The Urinal of Physick* are compositor's tricks to help in the justification of entire paragraphs – something that was considerably easier in the days before

Introduction

orthography and standardised spellings. Justification of paragraphs was not merely a cosmetic feature (as it is today). Early printers would be laying out discrete pieces of movable metal type into a square wooden frame and if the frame was not completely filled, the types might move under the action of the press and smudge the ink. In other words, each line of each paragraph had to extend fully from left to right, with the letters 'jammed' in the frame or the page would probably be unprintable.

One way for Renaissance printers to do this might have been by inserting blank spaces of suitable lengths between the words on each line, but this is not a satisfactory solution. The result is usually 'rivers' of blank space flowing down the page, which seriously interrupt reading and which was recognised as a problem from the very earliest days of printing. Hence the use of aggressive hyphenation, contracted words, diacritical marks and variant spellings of the same word, like the spelling of 'head' as hed (which has three letters), hedd (which has four), or hedde (which has five), all very useful when striving to obtain justification and spelling is not a problem. The compositor would use any or all of these tricks at will in order to obtain a solid block of text on each page.

FAULTS

The attentive reader will find some faults and errors in the pages of *The Urinal of Physick*, and, of course, no attempt has been made to indicate or remedy these in this facsimile reprint. Sometimes spelling mistakes occur despite the relaxed spelling conventions of the time, although these should more properly be regarded as typographical errors rather than mistakes in spelling as we understand the term today. An example is found on the first leaf *verso* of the dedication, line 22, where 'friudes' (friends) obviously has the letter n printed

Introduction

upside down. The word is repeated two lines down, with the n the right way up but with the i in the first instance replaced with y – 'fryndes'. There are a number of other instances in the text where either n or u have been printed upside down, rendering the resultant word, often with a variant spelling anyway, very strange-looking indeed. Another example of a spelling mistake is on leaf 31r, line 5, where 'strenght' (strength) obviously has the letters h and t transposed. When these and other typographical errors are encountered in this book, remember that they occur in the original printing and are faithfully reproduced in this facsimile reprint.

THE TITLE

The title of this book may seem strange to modern readers, even when acknowledging it as a medical textbook. However, the word 'urinal' did not have the same meaning in Recorde's time as it does today. Sometimes referred to by the Latin term 'matula', a urinal was a glass vessel specifically designed for the examination of urine in order to diagnose and treat illnesses. Many illustrations of contemporary physicians portray them holding a urinal, as on the title page of this book. According to Recorde '...as touching the urinal, it should be of pure clear glass, not thick nor green in colour, without blots or spots in it, not flat in the bottom, nor too wide in the neck, but widest in the middle and narrow still toward both the ends, like the fashion commonly of an egg, or of a very bladder being measurably blown (for the urinal should represent the bladder of a man) and so shall everything be seen in his due place and colour, if neither the grossness of the urinal, nor the colour, nor spots shall let the true sight of the colour, and substance of the urine, and the contents of it, neither the disform fashion of the urinal shall alter the regions or rooms of the urine.' That is, a good urinal

Introduction

should not alter or distort the appearance of the urine within it, and it should allow the contents to be viewed by the physician as though still in the bladder.

It is interesting to note that the physician in the title page illustration holds another tool of his trade in his right hand – an astrolabe. This would be used for astrological purposes, to view the stars and the zodiac in order to determine the most propitious times for treatment.

SOURCES

Readers wanting to know more about Robert Recorde should consult the following:

For an easily accessible biography visit the MacTutor History of Mathematics, 'Robert Recorde', [online]
http://www-history.mcs.st-andrews.ac.uk/Biographies/Recorde.html.

Written sources are:

Stephen Johnston, 'Recorde, Robert (c1512–1558)' *Oxford Dictionary of National Biography*, Oxford University Press, 2004.

Information about Robert Recorde's famous series of mathematical books can be found in:

Howell Lloyd, 'Famous in the Field of Number and Measure: Robert Record, Renaissance Mathematician', *Welsh History Review*, Vol. 2 (2000), pp. 254-282.

William Barr, 'A World View of Robert Recorde: A Brief Study of Tudor Cosmology, *Albion: A Quarterly Journal Concerned with British Studies*, Vol. 1, No. 1 (1969), pp. 1-9.

Joy B. Easton, 'The Early Editions of Robert Recorde's Ground of Artes', *Isis*, Vol. 58, No. 1 (Winter 1967), pp. 515-532.

Joy B. Easton, 'On the date of Robert Recorde's birth', *Isis*, Vol. 57, No. 1 (Spring 1966), p. 121.

Margaret E. Baron, 'A Note on Robert Recorde and the Dienes Blocks', *The Mathematical Gazette*, Vol. 50, No 374 (Dec 1966), pp. 363-369.

Louise Diehl Patterson, 'Recorde's Cosmography, 1556', *Isis*, Vol. 42, No. 3 (Oct 1951), pp. 208-218.

E.R. Sleight, 'Early English Arithmetics', *National Mathematics Magazine*, Vol. 16, No. 4 (Jan 1942), pp. 198-215 and Vol. 16 No. 5 (Feb 1942), pp. 243-251.

Francis R. Johnson & Stanford V. Larkey, 'Robert Recorde's Mathematical Teaching and the Anti-Aristotelian Movement', *The Huntingdon Library Bulletin*, No. 7 (Apr 1935), pp. 59-87.

David Eugene Smith & Frances Marguerite Clarke, 'New Light on Robert Recorde', *Isis*, Vol. 8, No. 1 (Feb 1926), pp. 50-70.

David Eugene Smith, 'New Information Respecting Robert Recorde', *The American Mathematical Monthly*, Vol. 28, No. 8/9 (Aug–Sep 1921), pp. 296-300.

Frank V. Morley, 'Finis Coronat Opus', *The Scientific Monthly*, Vol. 10, No. 3 (Mar 1920), pp. 306-308.

HERE BEGINS
THE
URINAL OF PHYSICK

The Vrinal
of Physick.

Compoſed by Mayſter
ROBERT RECORDE:
Doctor of Phyſicke.

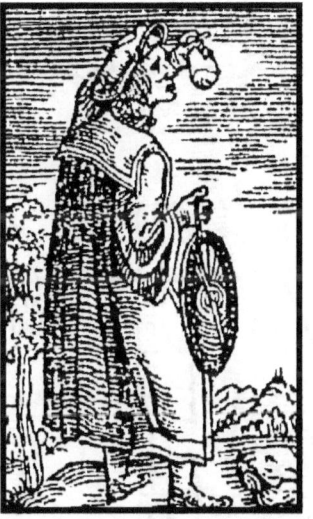

1 5   4 7.

Impꝛinted at London by Reynolde
Wolfe.
Cum priuilegio ad imprimendum ſolum.

An admonition to the Readers.

Reade all, or leaue all,
So am I perfecte and steddye.
To reade parte and leaue parte,
Ys to plucke ỹ lymmes frõ the bodie.

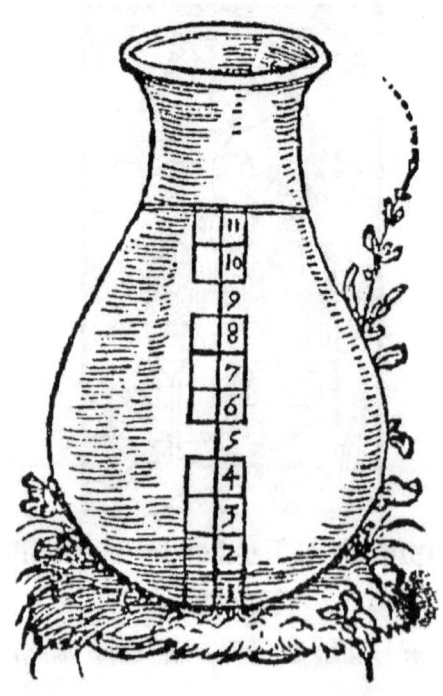

⁋ To the Wardens & company
of the Surgians in Lon=
don, Robert Recorde,
Doctor of Physicke,
wyssheth health.

WHen I cōsyder with my selfe,
what daunger he doth enter
that doth ought enterpryse,
which vnto mēnes syghte and hearing
shall cum : And on the other syde, how
quycke syghted most folke ar in other
mennes actes, and how prone to con=
troll, correcte and rebuke all mennes
doynges saue their owne : me thinkith
a man can not be to circumspecte, in a=
uoydyng all iust causes of reproche &
blame. Yet, syth there can be nothyng
so well done, but sum body agaynst hit
wyl rayle & iest, there is none otherway
to auoyde all soche tautes : but to lyue
ydle, & to meddle w̄ nothyng. so that I
may, as it semeth iustely thus cōclude :

    Syth it is so
    Procured by kynde,
    What one can do
    By wytte & mynde,
    An nother therto
              A.ij.   Sum

Sum faulte wyll fynde :
Yea lesse oz mo
Shall not him blynde.
Better it is,
Thy penne to refrayne,
Then often this
To moue disdayne,
Thou shalte not mysse,
But feele sum payne.
If thou loue blysse,
Therfoze abstayne.

But yet agayne consyderyng with my selfe, that if euery man shulde thus auoyde mennes tauntes, and refrayne too vtter truthe, foz feare of mennes checkes, then shulde the hole wozlde wander in ignozaunte : and feele all the euyls that of it may ensew.

Knowyng also that no man is bozne foz his owne singuler cõmoditie, & pzi= uate pzofyte : but that he ought to serue partely his parētis, partely his friēdes & partely his coūtrye : so that he is not wozthy to haue other parētes, fryndes, other coūtrye, that wyll refrayne to do them good foz any manner occasyon, moche moze foz the bespe bzablyng of curyouse carpers, & fond mynded men.

so that

so that agayne I conclude w my selfe, though nott so semely as before, yet more iustly: that he that wyll be profytable to the comen welthe, must not regarde those currish stomakes, which cā do nothyng but barke & brall: but must esteme them as vnmete to be cōsiderid of a wyse man, and moch more vnmete to be answered vnto. This wysedome may we learne of stomachouse horses, whiche contemptuously passe by the barkynge of curres, without countynaūce of feare, or token of reuengyng. But yet herein must boldenesse be temperyd, that hyt leade vs nott to enterpryse rashly, the thynge that maye be iustly blamyd, of wyse and sober men. So harde a thyng is it to kepe a meane, that menny doo fall into one faulte, whyle they laboure to eschew another.

The way therefore to auoyde both, and namely this rasshe boldenesse, is wysely too ponder, what you take in hande, and not to enterpryse what so euer your fantasy shall leade you vnto.

And yet farther, not to trust to your owne wytte, when you haue duly (as you thīke) wayd yt w your owne selfe,

A.iij.   But

But to refer youre enterpryse with the iudgement of hit also vnto sum other discrete, sober, wyse & lerned persone: which both wyll and can iudge of hyt, as hyt is worthy. by whose auctoritie, if thy worke shall be confyrmed, then mayst thou be bolde to let it go openly abrode, without fearyng any mannes checkes. For wyse, sober, and learned men wyll not condemne, nor blame hastely that thyng, that a wyse, sober, and lerned man hath approued and a= lowed. And if any other shall be mo= ued for lacke peraduenture of lernyng and iudgement, to improue any parte of it, and the soner if he regarde not, or truste not vnto thy autoritie : yet the autoritie of the persone vnto whõ theu hast dedicate thy boke, may cause him to refrayne if he haue any discre= tion. But if he be not only vnlerned, but also shameles, so that he wyl blame that he percepueth not, & corecte that he knoweth not, and mysse interprete, that he vnderstandeth not : yea, or (as sum do) condempne that he neuer red : soche one and his sayenges, you maye safely neglecte. More regardynge the
allowyng

allowyng of one wyse man, then the a
gayn sayeng of a thousand soch men.
   This thyng consyderyd, moued me
to flee, not onely vnto one man his
counsell, whiche peraduenture myght
seme to erre with me in iudgement, &
the soner, if he dyd bere affectiõ to me:
but rather vnto the counsell of menny,
not only beyng now in lyfe, but chefely
of them, which though they be ded in
body, yet thorough their excellẽt wor=
kes, shall lyue for euer. With those (I
say) haue I consulted, and so nearely
haue I followed their counsels, that I
may rightly call this my wrytyng, ra=
ther their worke then myne. Wherby
I myght be bolde to thynke that no
men (which at least be worthye to be
called men) wyll go about to depraue
that thing, that is alowed of so menny
excellent clerkes, both Grekes & La=
tyns, besyde Arabitians & other. Yet
I know that sum there be (I dare not
call them men) which wyll seke in hit
none other thyng then what thei may
rail at. but as for soch mõsters I force
not what they say of me & my worke,
syth I know them to be of that sorte,
              A.iiij.   which

which delyte to depraue nature & hyr workes, yea I may say, euen the God of nature.

Now therfore to leaue them, whose malyce I nothyng regarde, & to resorte to you, whom I esteme as a company not onely sober, dyscrete and wyse, but also so honestly & ernestly affectyd towarde all good knowledge, namely, that which may be any helpe and furtheraunce to that necessary arte which you haue professed: that you wyll both kyndely & thankefully receyue the good wyll of him that hath taken any paynes for your helpe, in the sure vsynge of that excellente arte of Surgerye. whiche as hyt is an arte so necessarye, that without hyt, mannes health can not longe contynew: consyderyng the menny myshappes that chaunceth to men daily. so if any neglygēce or ignoraunce be espyed in any one minister of hit, by and by that faulte is improched to the contempte of the hole arte. For the better and more certayner vse therof, nothing is more necessary then the exacte knowledge in Anatomye, to thentent you maye perceyue the hole
course

courſe of the vaynes, with the lyke diſtribution of the Arteries ioyntly paſſyng with them: and namely in ſoche places wher blood is vſed to be drawẽ: that an Artery be not ſtrycken in ſtede of a vayne, & ſo daunger ſuccede in the ſtede of remedy. Agayne, the Muſkils and ſynowes whiche cauſe ſenſe & motion, often tymes be ſo hurte and cutte in menny men, that other ſence or moupng of the hurte parte, is loſt: which thynge if the Surgian do not know, & before hande make declaration thereof to the pacyent, it chaunceth often that the pacientes impute the faulte to ſurgery: and ſo are occaſyoned to ſlaunder that moſt neceſſarye arte, bycauſe they are not taught to perceyue the iuſt cauſe where it is.

Menny mo inconuenieces might wel be auoyded, & great comodities therby pcured, if ther wer ã exact boke drawẽ of Anatomy, w̃ the ſituation & vſe of euery parte: which thynge as J haue long mynded, ſo J entend ſhortly to accomplyſh, with goodly pictures aptely framed, if J may pceyue that you, for whoſe ſake J do it, wyll with as good
                      A.v.   wyll

wyll accepte it, as I ſhall dꝛaw it. And in the meane ceaſon, foꝛ a token of my good wyll, I cõmend to your cuſtody, & dedicate to your vſe this lytle boke, which though it be ſmall in volume, yet is not ſmall in cõmodytie. and conſyderyng that foꝛ you it is pꝛofytable, not onely as it is to all other men, but alſo moꝛe peculyer: in ſo moch as often tymes by the water, you may perceyue the myſoꝛder of your pacyentes, not onely in tranſgreſſynge ſoche oꝛder of dyete as you ſhall with thaduyſe of a Phyſition inioyne them, but alſo dyuerſe other myſoꝛders, in excerſyce and other lyke, which myght not onely be a hynderaunce to the greife that you haue in cure, but alſo be an occaſyon that the myſdemenour of the pacient, & the hynderaunce of health that cummeth of him ſelfe, be imputed to you, as it often doth chaunce.

 Furthermoꝛe, you may lerne by the ſyght of the water, to iudge whether there be in the body any abundance of coꝛrupte mater, which doth contynually, as it is oftẽ ſene, miniſter ſupfluous excrementes to the greued mẽber.
And

And so procure that mater by sum in=
warde medicyne, with the counsell of
sũ lerned Physitiõ to be remoued : that
it be not a long stay against your cure.
 Furthermore by the water may you
coniecture, how moch the payne of the
sore doth greue the pacyent, & whether
it be lyke to cast him into any Ague or
greuous cõuulsion. For that doth sun=
dry tymes happen, that an outwarde
sore may cause an Ague, by his fyrie
inflammation. which if it do follow,
and be not by wyse counsell in tyme re=
systed, it may breede to the farther in=
flammation of the sayde sore : and so
consequẽtly not only procede to a more
diffyculte state of cure, but also to tor=
ment the pacyent with such intollera=
ble payne, that moch slaunder may re=
downde to the Surgiã therby, though
his diligẽce deserue rather gret thanke
then blame.
 Menny thinges also ar there, wher=
by it may appere, that great & dyuerse
cõmodyties are to be getheryd in the
vse of Surgery, by the obseruyng and
due markyng of vrynes. Of all which
if I shuld wryte peculierly, it were suf=
fycient

ficiēt mater foꝛ a large boke. Wherfoꝛe
I wyll foꝛ this tyme say no moꝛe, but
only desyꝛe you w as louynge a mynde
to accept thys my paine, as I haue of
a good wyll taken it, foꝛ the cōmodytie
both of your companye, & alſo foꝛ the
pꝛofyte of the hole commyns . whiche
thynge if I maye well perceyue, there
shall not want any good wylle noꝛ yet
paynes in me to further your studyes,
& ſo helpe your laboures : in any ſoche
kynde of knowledge, as other I shall
thynke meete foꝛ your arte, other you
youre selfes shall be desyꝛouſe to haue
wꝛytten, and set furth, as moſt may be
to your cōmodytie and contentation.
which paynes I wyll the moꝛe gladly
take , to pꝛouoke you to refuſe ſoche
tryfelyng bokes, as are set furthe in to
great a nomber : and that rather foꝛ the
aduauntage of the Pꝛinter, then foꝛ
the furtheraunce of mannes health.
which bokes, though my truſt be that
moſt parte of your companye, of a iuſt
conſyderation doo refuſe as vayne and
diſceytefull : yet I can not chuſe but
thynke that ſum other of youre com=
pany, whiche are yonge and desyꝛouſe
of

of straunge experimentes, doo ouer=
moche credit, and followe to boldely.

And yf you be despzouse peraduen=
ture to knowe their names, consyde=
rynge that by nampynge them, I might
prouoke the myndes of sum men ra=
ther to malyce then to amendement:
I wyll lette theym passe tyll a nother
tyme, desyringe you to trust moast in
the meane ceason to Johan Uigo, that
good Surgyan: whiche as he is tran=
slate by the dilygent paynes of Bar=
tholmew Traheron, is moast surest
foz you to follow in the arte of surgery:
& in manner alone foz any other that
I know.

Howbehyt, in Physicke sum other
haue taken commendable paynes:
whose despze, as I iudge to be, to
pzofyte the commens, and to ayde the
vnlerned, so I trust they wyll fozesee
that there shall no faute escape theym,
that may any wayes cause erroure to
increase. But contrarye wayes wyll
so imploy their studies, that soch thyn=
ges as be nedefull in knowlege, maye
be so

be so truly & aptely set furth, that men shall pceyue them selfe well ayded there by. And in this doyng, as J wolde be glad to exhorte all lerned men, studiously to set furth soch necessary knowlege, so J wyll pmyse my helpe in the furtheraūce of the same: so that J mai vnderstād, that they which by it might enioy cōmodytie, are so desyrouse to receyue it, & glad also to study it, that the setters furth therof, may thynke their paynes well bestowed. And agayne, if there be soch discretiō shewed in the reding & vsyng the same, that it may not be thought more inconuenyence, then profyte to ensewe thereby. in whiche thing, as touchyng Surgery, your discreate cyrcumspection may helpe very moch. vnto which, as J do surely trust, so J thynke it vnnedefull to geue you any further admonition by this wrytyng, but with ernest affection, commytte you vnto God / whiche is the right enstructer of all true knowledge,

       Fare you well.

⁋ At my house in London.
8. Nouemb. 1547.

ℭ The preface.

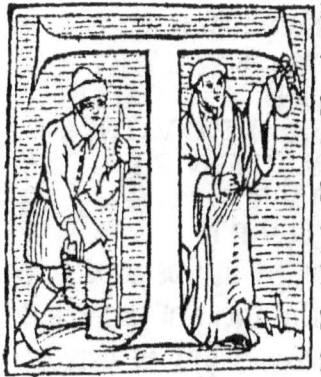

Though the vnsacyable gredynes of the couetouse men do mē ny & sundry wayps hurte, yet sũ waps it may do no lesse good, yf mē wyl not dysdayne (as they ought not) to vse hyt in soche sorte as I shall shew you.

The good vse of a couetous example.

But bicause that vnsaciabelnes is neuer satisfied, but besyde thowsandys of meanes inuentyd all redy to quēche ẏ͂ vnquencheable gredynes, hyt sekyth & findyth dayly newe and newe meanys vnnumerable, so that hyt were an infinyte laboure to declare them all. I wyll wyttingly & purposydly ouerpasse the greate rablement, only taking one generall sentence, whyche shall supply the stede of all the reste.

Vespasiane, one of the greate scole maisters of auarice, whiche could pyke oute profyte of euery thynge (yea,

A.j.   euen

THE PREFACE,

euyn of mennys vryne) taught his scolers (J mene ye hole courte of couetouse persons) thys lesson ensewynge:
LVCRE YS SWETE,
AND HATH A GOOD
SAVOVR, THOVGH
YT CVM OF VRY-
NE, DVRT, OR
ORDVRE.

Thys sentence, yf hyt be wythdrawẽ from the fylthy lucre of vnsaciable couetousnes, where in hyt is detestable, and employed rather to the dewe lucre of mãnys sustinaũce, then is hyt becum tolerable. But yf hyt be referryd to the necessary lucre of mannys helthe, then ys hyt greatly comẽndable. ℭ Jf there can be then any comõdite for mannys helthe, getheryd out of vryne (as there maye be muche) were it not a great rebuke vnto all mẽ that they shuld be found neglygente in sekynge of that thinge which shuld do good, both to them selfe and other? seynge the couetouse are so diligent in sekynge for that thinge, whiche shall profyt nother them selfe nor other? And the rebuke is so muche the greater

THE PREFACE, 2.

ter, if they shal be founde more slouth=
fuller in sekinge for this necessary cō=
moditie in a case so laudable, then are
the couetouse in a superfluouse despye
in a case so execrable.

But in as moch as this thinge (by re=
so it is not plainly set furth, is no lesse
difficult to be studied, thē it is necessa
rie to be vsed, the ignoraūt may haue
sum excuse, I therefore in the name of
many other, haue takē this paynes on *Ignoraūce*
me, to set forth this thinge so playnly, *set a syde.*
that ignoraūce can haue none excuse.

    But that no man shulde doubte of
the truthe of this treatyse, or of myne
entent in puttyng furth the same, ra=
ther in this our english tong, then any
other, I shall breefely shew reasons of
bothe.   Fyrst for the truthe of it I
wyll boldely speke, knowyng for cer=
tayne that no man that can iudge it,
wyll otherwayes other thynke or say
of it, but that it is as trew as mannes
knowlege can deuyse it. Namely, syth
it is wrytten accordyng to the myndes
of the most excellent wryters of Phy=
sicke, bothe of the Grekes and of the
           B.ij.   Latins

THE PREFACE,

Latyns. J meane Hippocrates, Galen, Aëtius, Aegineta, Philotheus, Theophilus, Actuarius: alſo Corneli' Celſus, Plinius, Cõſtantinus Africanus & Clementius Clementinus, with other mo. Conferryng alſo with theſe, Auicenna, Egidius, Polidamus and ſuche lyke: But with what temperance and moderation, they that ar lerned may perceyue. Theſe haue J folowed chefely in the Judicialles.

And in the vſe of medicine and dyſeaſes touchyng vrine, J haue ioyned with them, Dioſcorides, Quintus Serenus, Columella, Sext' Platonicus & dyuers other. Now if there be any man that douteth of the truth of thoſe wꝛiters in this thynge, J force nott though he doubt alſo of my truth in the ſame.

But now as touchyng myne entent in wꝛityng this treatiſe in the engliſh. *Thintent of* Though this cauſe might ſeme ſufficient to ſatiſfy many men ẏ J am an engliſh man, & therfore may moſt eaſely and plainly wꝛite in my natyue tonge rather then in any other: yet vnto thẽ that

Thintent of the autor.

THE PREFACE, 3.

that know the hardnes of the mater, this answer shuld seme vnlykely: conſiderig that it is moʒe harder to tranſlate into ſuche a tonge, wherein the arte hath not ben wʒitten befoʒe, then to wʒite in thoſe tonges that ar accuſtomed, and (as I might ſay) acquainted with the termes of the ſcience.

Nother is it ſo eaſy a thing (as ſum eaſy occupyed folke do thinke) to tranſlate well. Foʒ vnles that a man be able to perceyue not onely the woʒdes, but alſo the phraſe and kyndes of ſpeking of the tong, out of which he doth tranſlate, he ſhall not be well able to tranſlate. And if any man do not beleue me in this, I ſay no moʒe, but let him pʒoue it, and he ſhall ſo fynde it. I could ſhew furth here examples ſufficient, ſauying that I delyte not in blamīg other mēnes diligence, which we ſhuld rather commend, ſyth they dyd, after their abilitie, labour to pʒofyte many, yea the hole cōmunaltie.

To ouerpaſſe this, and to ſhew bʒefely the moſt vʒgent cauſes mouyng me to this enfoʒcement. I am ſure, there
are

THE PREFACE,

ar but few that euer sought coūsell for their helth, but they know that y͞e com̄me trade to attayne to the knowledge of the disease, is by y͞e Judicial of vrine, though not alone, yet as the principall. And lykewyse as there is not any thig so good, but the abuse of it may cause harme to ensew of the same: So this Judiciall of vrines, though it be a thyng hyghly to be regarded, yet if it be vsed rashly without comunicacion, or other sygnes knowen therewith, might cause (as it doth often) som error to be in the sentence of the Physicion, though he were right excellently learned: not so moche by the ignorāce of the physicion, as by lacke of knowledge in the pacient, which shuld enstructe the physicion in soche questiōs as he neded to demaunde of him: and not to looke that the physicion shuld tell him all thynges at the fyrst syght, more lyke a God then a man.

So that if there be any physicion so arrogaunte, that he wyll take vpon him to tell all thynges alone, & wyll not here the paciēt speke, specially not
knowyng

THE PREFACE, 4.

knowyng the partie before, neither se=
yng other sygnes but the onely vrine,
as I dare boldly pronounce that soch
a man is vnworthy to be called a phy=
sicion: So it shalbe good for all men,
not to trust to the iudgement of soche
one. For by soch mysuse in this thyng
hath not only moch harme chaunsed
vnto the pacientes, so that it hath ben
thoccasion of many mēnes death, but
also very moch reproche hath ensued
to the hole estate & ordre of physicions
and hath caused that excellent & most
necessary arte to be contempned, deri=
ded, and lytle set by.

To auoyde the more better this in=
conuenience, I haue writen this lytle
treatyse to all men in commen, that
they may lerne to haue sum knowlege
in their owne vrines, and therby may
be the better able to enstructe the phy=
sicion, in this thyng at the least, what
sorte of vrine they haue made from
tyme to tyme, syth the beginnyng of
their sycknes, and sumwhat before.
And also what sort of water they wer
wonte to make customably in their
    B.iiij.   health:

The vse of this booke.

THE PREFACE,

helth : so that if men wyll be diligent to marke their water in tyme of helth, they shall not only be able to enstruct y̆ physicion (as I haue sayd) but shuld be also able to perceyue the cause of the disease sumtymes before the grefe cum, & so by the counsell of sum discrete physicion, auoyde the sycknesse before it be fully entered : pea, and by dew markyng of their vrine, they shal perceiue from tyme to tyme, how they shall gouerne them selfes in meates & drinkes, in exercyse and rest, & lyke other thynges, so that thereby they may eschew both the diseases and also the causes of the same.

Now what a commoditie this may be to all men, and what thankes he hath deserued that hath taught this so great a commodytie to all men in generall, I remyt it to euery mannes owne iudgement.

And thus (as you may pceyue) I haue declared the causes of this my paynes takynge, to be for the profyte of the hole commens indifferently. How be it, if any meane learned phisicion shal

THE PREFACE, 5.

ſhal vſe it to his any lytle helpe in iud=
gement, I wyl not enuy him, but wy
be the gladder, the moꝛe nomber of mē
I perceyue to take pꝛofyt by it.

 I am ſure that the true iudiciall of
vꝛines, accoꝛdig to the mynde of Hip=
pocrates, Galen, and ſoch lyke, is ve=
ry harde, though not to excellent cler=
kes, yet to the meane ſoꝛte, partely by
reaſon that it is wꝛitten ſo diſperſedly
in their woꝛkes ⁊ not in any one boo=
ke peculyerly ⁊ ſufficiētly : and partely
by cauſe that ſundꝛie woꝛdes vſed in
the ſame (as in the reſt of phyſicke) ar
obſcure to them that haue not ben ex=
ercyſed (in maner) in all kyndes of ler
nynge, and that with the knowledge
of both the Greke and Latē tonges.
Therfoꝛe I truſt that this my paines
ſhalbe ſum helpe alſo to thē that lack
the exercyſe of ſoch ſtudy ⁊ knowlege.

 But bycauſe there is a cōmen ſay=
eng in the mouthes of many mē now
a dayes, that it is a pꝛofanyng of ler=
nyng, ⁊ a meanes to bꝛing it in to con=
tempte, ſo to ſet it foꝛth in the vulgar
tonge, that euery man indifferently
may

The difficulte of iudgement yn Vrine.

THE PREFACE,

T hanſwere vnto it.

may rede it & ſtudy it. To this I wyll bꝛefely anſwere, that this ſayeng is not only agaynſt many great learned mennes actes and examples, but alſo agaynſte manyfeſt reaſon : beſydes that it encludeth a pernicious kynde of coūſell. For if euery thyng ſhulde be put awaye, oꝛ lefte vndone, that e= uyll men coulde peruerte and vſe to an euyll purpoſe, ſo ſhulde we haue no good thyng remayne. meates & drin= kes muſt be taken away, bicauſe many abuſe it. And bycauſe euyll men do abuſe bothe eyes & tonges ſhal all men therfoꝛe plucke out their eyes & their tonges? Bycauſe many men do abuſe lawes and auctoꝛitie, ſhall men expell lawes & hygh powers? Many a wo= mā hath ben defiled vnder cloke of cō= feſſion, & ſhuld we therfoꝛe refuſe the good vſe that is in chꝛiſten confeſſion? Many euyl mē & heretikes haue miſſe enterpꝛeted goddes woꝛde, yet ought godes woꝛd neuertheles to be taught vulgarely to all men. Though Cardi= nalles & mōkes haue pꝛactiſed to poy= ſon men euē with the very ſacrament

of

THE PREFACE, 6.

of the aulter: yet no mã wyll be so mad therfore to eschew the vse of that blessed sacramẽt. And yet al this foloweth if men alow that commen sayeng aboue wꝛitten. better menes it were to set furth publykely, all that myght do good to y̓ publyke wealth, & straightly to punysh y̓ abusers of them, rather then to punysh good men & good thynges, bycause y̓ euyll men offende. It is a lyke erroꝛ to that soꝛte of doctrine, which condempned wyne as an euyll thyng, bycause that many were made dꝛonkẽ with it. ⁋ But to leue this, & to cum moꝛe particulerly to the mater What is lernyng vnlerned, oꝛ knowledge vnknowne? any thing els but a vayne name? Lernyng then encreseth most, when it is studyed of most: & lernyng then triumpheth most, when it hath most fauoꝛers & folowers. & then doth ygnoꝛaunce (lernynges enemye) reioyce most, when lernyng reygneth in fewest, and blyndnes ruleth most. so that then is lernyng most pꝛofaned, contempned and hated, when she hath most enemyes: that is to saye, when

most

THE PREFACE,

Plutarche his ſcentēce

moſt men ar ignozaunt : foz that olde ſayeng ſhal alwayes be trew. Lernyng hath none enemye, but the ygnozaūt.

Aſke that great clerke Plutarche what his mynd is in this : whether the Judiciall of helth be a mete thyng foz euery mā to ſtudy : and thou ſhalt here him anſwere : that ſhame it is foz men to obſerue the cryeng of crowes, and ſoche lyke thinges in beaſtes and byz= des, whereby men iudge chaūge of we= thers, and to be negligent in marking mocions within them ſelfe, and alte= rations pzeparyng vnto ſycknes : yea he requyzeth ſo exacte knowlege in e= uery man appteinyng vnto helth, that he noteth it foz a great rebuke, & cal= leth it vnſenſyblenes in a man, if he be ſo ignozaunt that he ſhal nede to aſke of ẏ Phyſicion, what meates are beſt foz him . And to aſke, what meates ſhall beſt diſgeſt in him, is as vncumly a queſtion (ſayth he) as to aſke, what meates ar ſwete, ſower, oz bytter, and ſoche lyke. yea beyond all this, he re= quyzeth in euery man the knowledge of his owne pulſe, which is a thyng
harder

THE PREFACE, 7.

harder then ẏ iudicial of vrines. Now if you requyre eraples, the hole worlde is full of them. They that wrote in Greke, wrote in their owne vulgare tong: & so dyd they that wrote in Latyn, write in their commen speche. Besydes that, haue we not infinite eraples of lerned mē in Germany, Fraūce & Spayne, which wrote of Physike in their own tōge? yea, is not our own England full of eraples? How many bokes of practyses, how many Herballes & other lyke bokes of Physicke hath there ben put furth many yeres passed? And yet vnto this day do not lerned wyttes sleepe. How moch is all England bounde to that worthye knyght, & lerned clerke, sẏr Thomas Elyote, whiche tooke the paynes to buylde a castell of helth for all Englishmen (besydes many other goodly bokes that he hath put furth in the vulgare tong) wherby a man may lerne bothe to gouerne him self so, that though he escape not all sycknesses quyte, yet he shall eschew the great daungers of them. England may reioyce

Examples of wryters in the vulgare tonge.

Sir Thomas Elyot.

THE PREFACE,

ioyce of foch a knyght: yea, England hath to few that foloweth foch example. But if Englande hadd as many welwyllyng doers, as fhe hath cruell and fpytefull difdayners, then were England the flower of al Realmes in the worlde.

Now wyll I leue this and drawe nerer to my purpofe, and wyll defyre all men that fhall rede this booke paciently to bere with my boldenes, and thankefully to receiue my good mynd. And if there fhalbe found in this boke or in any other that I fhall put furth any fmall error or ouerfyght (for great errors I dare fay there fhalbe none) I fhal defyre al them that fhall fo fynd or thynke, to aduertyfe me therof by worde or wrytyng, and I fhalbe redy not only to render condygne thankes, but alfo, other to amende dewly, that fhalbe thought a myffe, or els to yelde refonable lernyng for the profe of the fame. ❡ And now to make an ende I wyll defyre euery man fobrely & difcretely to vfe this my booke, not abufyng it to the tauntyng or checking of other

The exhortation to the Reader.

THE PREFACE, 8.

other men : nor to gether boldenes & trust in their owne knowlege, further then they ought.

And lyke wayes I shall exhorte all men, not to mocke and gest with any Physicion (as sum lyght wyttes do) temptyng them with Beastes stale in stede of mēnes Urine : other bryng= yng to them mēnes water for womēs, and soch other lyke thynges. For in this doyng they deceiue not the Phy= sicion but themself. For a mānes wa= ter to be lyke a womans, it nede seme no straūge thyng. How be it, agayne, there is notable difference, in so moch that that water which in a man decla= reth certayne helth, if it were a wo= mans, might declare sum disease. and lyke wayes that that in a woman pre= tendeth helth, if it were a mans wa= ter, it mought betoken syckenes. And if a mans water and womans be lyke and betoken both diseases, those dis= eases may be dyuerse, and not one.

yea .ii. mēnes waters beyng both lyke shall not declare alwayes one grefe, ex cepte they agree also in age, dyet, ex=
ercyse

THE PREFACE,

ercyſe and lyke other thynges.

Alſo that a beaſtes water may be lyke a mannes (the mannes ſyckneſſe beyng thereafter) Hippocrates wyt=neſſeth, and experience techeth, as I ſhall declare hereafter. Therfore if you ſeke the pacyentes health, looke that you receue the vrine dilygently & as ſone as you can preſent it to the Phyſiciõ, and be diligent to enſtruct him in all thynges that you can, and that he ſhall nede to aſke. And ſo no doubte, you ſhall recepue great commoditie of that arte, to the helth of man, and the glory of God, which hath geuen ſoch knowledge vnto man.

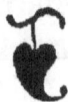

¶ Of the diuision & ordre of this booke. The fyrst Chapiter.

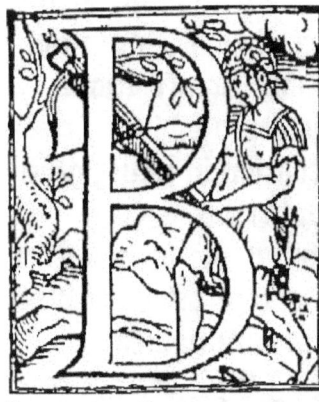

Bcause that nothynge done vnorderly cann be well vnderstanded of the reders, & euery thige the better ordre it hathe, ỹ beter it may be vnderstand, and also moche more easely be remembred, when the ordre of it is well and certenly knowne. I haue therfore digested this boke into a certayne and orderly processe, which I shall here set furthe to thentent that you may rede, as it were in grosse, the whole booke, and thereby kepe it the better in remembraunce.

The summe of this boke

i. Fyrst therfore I wyll declare the nature of vrine, what it is, and how it is engendred within man, and how it passeth furth from man.

ij. Secte, of the ordre of receuyng it with vessell dew. And of the tyme and place meete to conspdre it.

C.j. Thirdly

THE IVDICIAL

Thyrdly, how many thynges ar to be cōsidred in vrin : & how many ways they may be altered in a helthful man.

Fourthly, what significations & tokens may be gethered of vrine, concernyng any alteration in man, other paste, or present, or to cum.

Fyfthly, to what vse in medicine vrine may serue, and of other good vses of it to mannes commoditie.

And last of all, I wyll declare certayne diseases touchyng vrine, which other let it, or cause it to voyde vnwyllyngly : with the medicines and remedies meete for the same.

How vrine is engendred in Man, and how it passeth furth. The .2. Chapter.

As vnto them that ar lerned, & know by the art of Anatomy the situation of the partes of man, and the naturall offyce of euery parte, it is esye ynough to perceue the original generation and cause of vrine without any example, so vnto theym that nother knowe the situation nor offyces

OF VRINE. 10.

offices, no nother yet the names of the partes of mannes bodye, it is scarse possyble to make them to perceue the generacion of vrine without sum sensible example. But bycause it is very harde to fynde an artificiall example, whiche can a lone duly expresse this worke of nature, I wyll vse therfore an example of a natural worke, which shall expresse in menny poyntes this thyng, though not in all: for soche can there none be, but the thyng it selfe.
And in as moche as this example is not easy to be vnderstand of all men, though the most parte do now a daies partely know it by experience of fyndyng springes of waters. I wyll fyrst propose an artificial example, to make the other bothe ẙ beter to be perceued

It is daily sene in distillyng of waters, that the temperate heate of the fyer doth seperate the purest parte of the iuce frõ the herbes, & also from the grosser iuce. This by natural lightnes is drawen into the hed of the stillatory wher by the coldenesse of the helmet it is made sumwhat grosser, & so thorow

An exãple of ſtillyng.

C.ij. naturall

THE IVDICIAL

Thoriginal cause of sprynges.

naturall heate descendeth and passeth furthe by the pype of the stillatory. And as the arte of man vseth to make this water, so doth nature vse to make the water of sprynges, wherof cum all ryuers, stremes and flouddes, excepte the see. For seyng the erth is not parfectly sounde and thycke of substance, as stones and sum wooddes appereth to be, but is hollow and full of holes as you se that corke is: so that the ayer which by his subtylnes perseth euery neuer so lytle a hole, entreth & fylleth this hollownes, nature so ledyng it, bycause no place shulde be emptye / in whiche place by the coldenesse of the erth, the ayer is turned into water, as you may se in walles and pyllers of stone, namely of marble, how the coldnesse of the stone turneth the ayer into water & hangeth full of drops, which sum tyme tryckle downe a pace, as if they dyd swete. So when the erth hath turned the ayer thus into water, then doth it dropp downe & gethereth to gether, and so runneth out as it can fynde or prepare way. As longe therfore

OF VRINE   II.

foze as there is hollowneſſe in that place, with ſoche ſozte of coldeneſſe, & none other let, the ſpzing of water ſhal neuer ceaſe. But and if the way by any menes be ſtopped, then the water toz= moyleth and labozeth, other to expell that let, oz to make a new way.

Now this water beynge thus engen= dzed of the ayer, which hath no taſte, is alſo naturally without all taſte / but the taſt that it hath, is the taſte of the vaynes of erth oz metall, by which it doth rūne. And that is the cauſe that ſum waters are ſweete, & ſum ſower, ſum freſh, and ſum ſalte, & other ways dyuerſely tayſted: ſum alſo ar hotte & ſum colde, and with other lyke quali= ties endued, accozdyng to the ground wherby it paſſeth: But of this I wyll not now ſpeke, bicauſe I haue appoin ted foz it a peculyer treatyſe, if God graunte me tyme. Onely this I ſay now, that a man that is experte, can by ẏ colour, taſte, and other qualities of the water, which he ſeyth, tel what vaynes of earthe oz mettalles is in that place whence that water cūmeth

The cauſes of diuerſite in taſte of Water.

C iij.   though

THE IVDICIAL

though he see it not.

And this water is expelled out of his fyrst place as vnprofytable there to remayne / and yet when it is cum furth thence, it is good for dyuerse & sundry vses. Thus may we thynke of the generation & vse of vrine or mans water. It shall not nede here to reken exactly the places, causes & thordre of the .iij. cõcoctions which go before the generation of vrine / but it shall suffyce to tell brefely, that of the meate & the drynke together concocted in the stomake, is made rude bloude (if I may so cal it) which rude bloud is wrought agayn and made more perfecter in the lyuer : and thyrdly yet more purifyed in the hollow vayne / where the vrine is separate frõ it, as whey frõ mylke : but yet may not exactly be called vrine tyll it cum into the raynes (or kydnes) which draw it out of the hollow vayn by a certayne naturall power restyng in them / And then doth the raynes (or kydneys) alter it parfectely into vrine, as the coldenes of the ground turneth ayer into water. But you must take
this

The generation of vrin

OF VRINE 12.

this comparison oz similitude too be spoken of the alteration it self & not of the cause. Now whan vzine is this made, lyke to the facyon of water, as I sayde, then as the water passeth furth from his fyzst place, by pisshewes outwarde, so doth the vzine descende from the raynes by certayne vaynes (as it were) called water pypes, and runneth into the bladder: frõ whence at due tymes, it is expelled furth if the way be not let. So that you may com̅pare the raynes to y̅ hed of a cũdyte: the water pypes, to the cũdyte pypes: the bladder, too the cundyte: and the shafte to the cocke of the cundyte.

And further as the water doth de̅clare by taste & colour, the qualyties of the erth, oz vaynes of metall, wher̅by it runneth and from whence it cum meth: so the vzine by coloure & othez wayes, declareth of what sorte the pla ces that it cũmeth thozow, & humozs that it cummeth from, are affected.

And yet not onely serueth foz this, but also as the water though it depte from the erth, as superfluous in that place, yet in other places and to other

THE IVDICIALL

purposes it is greatly profytable. So the vrine, though it be expelled as a superfluous excrement, yet besyde this commodytie of iudgement, whiche it geueth of the partes that it cummeth frõ, it doth also serue for the dyuerse vses in medicine, and other good commodyties: of which both I wyll anon orderly wryte, after I haue declared certayne thinges appertaining to the dew iudgement of it.

Of the Instrument and partes by which Uryne is engendred and passeth, marke this fygure folowyng.

OF VRINE. 13.

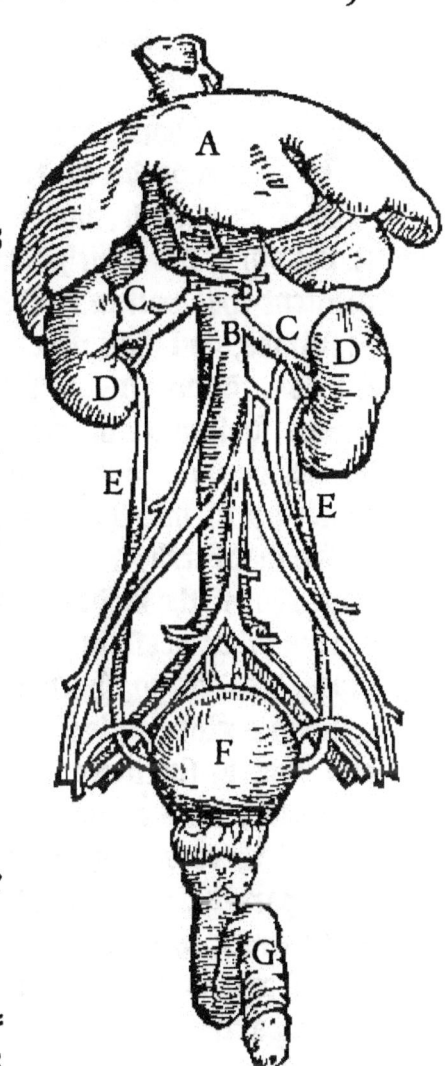

A. is the lyuer.

B. the ho low vaine.

C. vaynes by whiche the reanes do draw ẏ vrine, and therfore be called suck= yng vaynes

D. ẏ renes

E. the wa ter pypes.

F. is the bladder.

G. ẏ spou te of the yar de.

All the o= ther partes besyde, appertaine to Generation and seede.

Cv.   What

THE IVDICIAL

What vrine is, and what tokens it geueth in generall. The .3. Chapiter.

YOU haue herde now how vrine is engendered, from whence it cummeth, and by what places it passeth, the which thynges all to thentent that you may the better kepe in mynde, you shall note this shorte diffinicion. Urine is the superfluitie or wheye substaunce of the bloude in the hollow vayne, coueyed by the renes & water pypes into the bladder.

The diffinicion of V=ryne.

So that hereby you may plainly perceue, that if the bloode be pure & clene, & none other grefe in the renes, water pipes, bladder, nor shafte: then shal the vrine so declare it, beyng also parfecte and pure in substance and coloure and al other tokens accordyng to the same But if there be any greefe in any of those partes, or the blood corrupte by any menes, then shal the vrine declare certen tokens of the same, as I shall anone particulerly expresse. But fyrst it shalbe necessary to instruct you of the vessel, place & tyme meete to iudge vrine, & of the maner of receupng it.

Of

OF VRINE. 14.

Of the forme of the Vrynall, and of place and tyme meete to iudge vryne, and how it shuld be receued. The .4. chapiter.

That vrine shuld be kepte to see, which is firſt made after mydnyght comenly, oꝛ namely when the pacient hath ſlept loṅg. but you muſt take heede (whether the pacient be mã oꝛ woman) that they make not their vrine in a nother veſſell fyꝛſt (as many vſe to do) & then powꝛe it into the vrinall when it is ſetled, foꝛ that cauſeth moch deceite & errroꝛ in the iudgement of it. And if that the pacyent can not well make it in the vꝛinall, other by wekeneſſe, oꝛ any other cauſe, the n let them make it in an other veſſell, but ſe that it be clene & dꝛy: & as ſone as the water is made, powꝛe it furth ſtreight wayes into the vꝛinall all together, & leue no parte of it out, as ſum curious folke do vſe to put the clere parte only into the vꝛinall & caſt a way the dꝛegges: as though it ſtode not with their honeſty to bꝛynge ſoche foule gere to the Phyſicion, other of any lyke folyſh mynd. Powꝛe it therfoꝛe in wholly, and let not the vꝛinall ſtand open,

The order to receyue vryne.

THE IVDICIALL

namely in a dusty place, but stopp it close to a gloue or other lether, & not with cloth, paper, nor hey, and let it be brought to the Physicion within vj. howers at the furdest: for after that tyme it can not well be iudged.

The vrinal.   Now as touchyng the Vrinall, it shulde be of pure clere glasse, not thyck nor greene in colour, without blottes or spottes in it, not flat in the bottom, nor to wyde in the necke, but widest in the myddell and narrow styll towarde bothe the endes, lyke the facyon commenly of an egg, or of a very bladder beyng mesurably blowen (for the vrinal shuld represet the bladder of a mã) and so shall euery thyng be sene in his dew place and coloure / if nother the grossenes of the vrinal, nother the colour, nor spottes shal let the true syght of the colour, and substaunce of the vryne, and the contentes of it / nother the dyfforme facyon of the vrinall shal alter the regiõs or romes of the vrine.

The place.   Lyke wayes concernynge the place meete to behold vrines / you must loke that it be nother to darke, so that your
                                            syght

OF VRINE 15.

sight shuld not discerne parfectly other the coloure, substaunce or contentes for lacke of lyght: nother yet that your syght be likeways deceued, if the place be to lyght, as in open lyght or bemes of the sunne.

Besydes this also must ye marke the tyme dew to behold vrines: but bycause there can no one tyme be assygned certayne and exacte to iudge all partes of it, I wyll breefely shew he order of the thynges to be consydered in their tyme. *The tyme.*

Fyrst, when the vrine is made, whyle it is yet sumwhat hotte, you shall consyder the coloure of it: for that may best be descerned then, and lykewayes the thycknes of the substaunce of it: which if it be meane, shall then be best sene. All other thynges, as the bubles, & the contentes shalbe best iudged sumwhat after when the vrine is sumwhat cooled, and they be duly setled in their vpper places.

How many thynges ar to be consydered in Vryne, The 5. Chapiter.

Now leuyng this as a breefe instruction, of the generation of the water or vrine, and of the maner of re=

TEE IVDICIAL

of receuyng it in veſſels due, with tyme and place meete to conſyder it. I wyll particulerly declare how many thinges ar to be conſydered in it, which ar commenly named .iiij. that is the ſubſtance, the colour, the quantytie, and the contentes: and the ſauoure thereto may be added as the fyfte: to the whiche .v. if you ſhall ioyne ſtablenes & order as .ij. accidētes cōmen to the firſt .iiij. thinges but yet no leſſe to be cōſidered then thei, then ſhall you iudge the moꝛe certenly.

Stablenes

Vnſtable-neſſe.

Order.

Stableneſſe is called, when the vꝛine continueth certen dayes together of one ſoꝛte. And if it alter euery day, then is that called vnſtableneſſe oꝛ chaungeableneſſe, to which thyng oꝛdꝛe doth appertayne: Foꝛ oꝛdꝛe is the folowyng of one thyng after an other, as blacke coloured vꝛine after whyte, grene, oꝛ pale. I meane not, bycauſe that ſo it ought to folow, but onely that you muſt obſerue how it doth follow. Foꝛ blacke vꝛine doth nott ſynify the ſame, if it follow after grene vꝛine, as it doth, if it follow after white vꝛine: ſo that the oꝛdꝛe ought alſo to be marked..

But

OF VRINE. 16.

But now to retourne to the .iiij. fyrste thynges. Substaunce is called in vrine, the vrine it selfe in respecte of the thyknesse or thynnesse of it: so that there ar .iij. sortes of substance in vrine: thicke thynne, and meane. Thynne substance is called, when you may perceue wel the ioyntes of your fyngers through the vryne. And contrary wayes it is called thycke, when you can nott well see your fyngers through it: and that that is in the myddle betweene extreeme thycke & extreme thynne, is called, meane.

 Colours ar dyuerse, but the principal are these .vj. whyte, pale, flaxen, yellow, red, and blacke. And all the other coloures ar contayned vnder these .vj. As vnder whyte, ar contayned clere as cristall, whyte as snow, & pure as water which .iij. are lyght whytes. Then are there other .iij. more darker, as mylke whyte, clere lyke horne, and grey. After whyte, followeth pale coloure, & then flaxen, after it followeth palew, & then yellow, which may be called goldẽ, for it is the coloure of pure golde. After it followeth lyght saffren, & then saffron.

Substaũce

Thynne.

Thycke.

Meane.
Coloures.

Light white as Cristal=lyne. snowy Watery.
Darke whytes / as milke white horny. gray.
Pale/Flaxẽ
Palew /ye=low.
Lyght safrõ

THE IVDICIALL

Safferne colour.
Claret co=lour.
Red.
Crymſyn.
Purple.
Blew.
Greene.
Oylye.
Aſh colour
Blacke.

ſaffren, then claret coloure, & then redd: after it crymſyn, and then purple, and then blew. Then is there grene of dy=uerſe kyndes: as light græne, grene as graſſe, ſtarke grene, and darke grene.

There are alſo oyle coloures (that is popigey grene) of .iij. ſortes, as of grene: lyght oylye, ſtarke oylye, & darke oylye. After theſe is there aſſh coloure, lyke vn to led: and after it (as laſt of all) cũmeth blacke, & theſe be the chefe coloures.

Quantytie

Now as touching quantitie, it is alſo in .iij. ſortes, moche, lytle, and meane.

Moche.
Lytle.
Meane.

Then is it called moche quantytie, whẽ it excedeth the meaſure of a mans drin=kyng: and then is it called lytle, when a man pyſſeth leſſe then he drinketh. And ỹ is meane, when a mannes pyſ=yng and his drinkyng is of lyke quan=tytie. Al this muſt be conſidered by dew proporcion.

Contentes
Sedyment
Sublation
Cloude.

The contentes ar al thin=ges in the water, that be of another mat ter and ſubſtaunce particulerly, then is the vrine: as the ſedyment or grounde, the ſublacion or ſwymme, & the cloude. To theſe ar added other dyfforme cõten tes, lyke berys, lyke huſkys, lyke bran,

and

OF VRINE. 17.

and soch other. And also the crowne of the vrine, with the bubbyls, and other thynges swymmyng on the top of it.

   For the better vnderstandyng of these contentes, you must note, that the whole vrine from the top to the bottome, is deuyded commenly into .iij. romes or regions. The lowermost is the region of the grounde or sedyment : so that the groundes or sedymentes are the contentes that occupy the lowermost region : or yet more properlye the sedymente is called a certen substance of grosser mater then is the vrin, lyke to a quātytie of very watery flewme, which fleteth a lytel aboue the bottom of the vrine : but if it be so lyght, that it swym in the myddle region of the vrine, then is it called the sublation or swym. And if it be yet more lyghter, so that it doth fleete in the highest parte of the vrine, then is it called a cloude : whereby you may perceue that the grounde, the swym, and the cloude, are but one thyng in substance, & dyffer only by lyghtnes and heste, and taketh his name accordyng to the region that it occuppeth. But yet agayne note that

Grounde
Sedyment

Sublation
Swymme

Cloude

        D.j.   euery

THE IVDICIAL

euery one of the .iij. regions is farther deuided into other partes also, wherby you may know exactly how far all contetēs differ from the iust roume of their regiō: so that the whole vrine must be deuyded into a xj. iust partes, of which the nether region occupieth .iiij. the .v. is the voyde roome bytweene that and the myddle region, which conteineth .iij. moꝛe. that is to say, the syxte, seuenth and eyght. And then the nyenth is a voyde roume betweene the myddle regyon and the hyghest : which hyghest regyon, conteyneth the other two partes that remaine, that is the tenth & the leuenth, as this Fygure sheweth whyche here after folowyth.

About

OF VRINE.   18.

Aboue these iij. regions, about the very brin= ke of the vrin you may see a certen rynge as it were go yng about, & that is called the crowne. Highest of al thynges in the vrine are the bubbels, which other go about with the ryng on= ly, or els fleete in the myddell of the vrin only, or els bothe. Yea, sumtyme they couer all the whole topp of the vryne. Besyde these is there often tymes as it were a flotes, or fattynes on the topp, and sumtymes certayne spottes onely which are lyke to droppes of oyle. And these commenly ar the whole contentes. For as for grauell or stone, or any lyke thyng is contepned vnder the name of

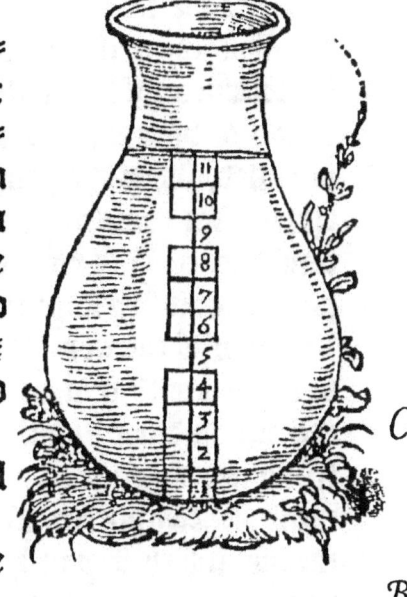

Crowne.

Bubles.

Fattyneſſe.

D.ij.   dyfforme

THE IVDICIAL

dyfforme contentes. You shall also vnderstande that in the contētes must the substaunce, the quantyte & coloure be obserued. The substaunce is other equall or vnequall. Equall substaunce is called, when the grounde, swym or cloude (for to them apparteyneth this consyderation) is not tattered and dispersed, but iustly knyt together.

Substaūce.
Equall.

Unequal is cōtrary, when it is thynne in one parte then in another, or flyttered out, and not suantly and vniformly ioyned together. The quantyte must be consydered in respecte to a meane, which if you know well, then may you soone iudge that to be ouer moche, that is more then it: and that to be to lyttle, that is lesse then it. But this meane quantyte must you lerne of a parsyte whole water, & best by the teching of sum good physicion. Of coloures I haue spoken before sufficiently for their varyetie.

Vnequall.

Quantytie

What a parsyte Vryne is, and also how many wayes all partes of the vryne may be altered in a helthfull man.
The .6. Chapiter.

Now

OF VRINE. 19.

Now that you know the differēce of soche thynges that ought to be cōsidered in vrine, before you shall lerne by consyderacion of them, to iudge of the parsone that made it, how he is dysposed in his bodye: you must fyrst know how many wayes the partes of the vrine may be chaunged in a helthfull man. For the better vnderstandyng of the which thyng, and of all that shalbe seyd hereafter, I wyl fyrst defyne what a parfecte whole vryne is: which as it betokeneth no grese in it selfe, so is it a trew rule to examyne all other vrines by that are not hole, but declare in them sum greese.

A parfyte hole vrine is meane in substaūce, and in quantyte, and in colour palew, or partle saffren, with a whyte grounde, duly knyt, and stable, without bubles and other euyll contentes. So that this parfyte hole vrine declareth the dyfference of al other vrines: For euery vrine the more it a greyth with this, the better it is: & the more it dyffereth from this, the worse it is, as I shall anone partyculerly declare.

Galen. li .8. capi .12. de Crisibus.

D.iij. And

THE IVDICIALL

And here you must marke that this parfecte hole vrine is not only ta=ken of a parfect hole man, but also of the lustyest tyme of mānes age, that is at .xxx. yeres: or more largely, betwene xxv. and .xxxv. For in euery age doth the vrine alter, as you shal here by & by

The dyfference of Vryne by age in men.

Chyldren.

Galen .2. prefag. Hippocra, 33.
Yong men.

Men.

Age.

The vrine of Chyldren differeth but lyttle in colour from palew or light saffren, and in substaunce it sumwhat excedeth in thyckenesse the substaunce of young mennes vrine, & hath moche grounde in it: And the more they doo grow in age, the hygher waxeth the coloure, the substaunce the thynner, & the lesse is the grounde. And therfore when age is most freshest, the colour is palew (so that the vrine of florishyng youth or parfyte manhod, is pallew or lyght saffren) and there resteth and goeth no hygher, and the grownde of it is meane: But now after that tyme, the more age encreseth & youth decay=eth, the more the colour chaūgeth from pallew toward whyte, & the grownde waxeth

OF VRINE 20.

waxeth lesser & darker: so that the v=
ryne of Olde men is thynne & whyte,
w lytle grouðde, enclinĩg vnto crudytie

Of the vryne of Women by age.

The vrine of women which ar tem= **Women.**
perate, in health & in their flourish=
yng youth, doth declyne sumwhat frõ
palew, & lyght saffren toward whyte,
and the substaũce is in maner thynne:
but it hath moꝛe grounde then mẽnes
vrine. Now all thei that be vnder this *Yong wo=*
flourishing age, the yonger thei be, the *men,*
whyter coloured is their vrine, & the
moꝛe grounde it hath: and if they be
elder, the moꝛe aged they ar, the why= *Aged wo=*
ter also is their vrine, but the grounde *men.*
is euer lesse & lesse. And thys you may
se how both diuersytie of age, & dyuer=
sitie also of kynd oꝛ sexe causeth altera
tion in vrine without chaũge of helth:
foꝛ you must vnderstand all these ages
with parfyte helth.

*The diuersytie of vrynes accordyng to
the tymes of the yere.*

D.iiij.   Euen

THE IVDICIAL

Spryng

Euen as diuersytie of ages altereth vrine, so doth the tymes of the yere: For the more that y̓ sprĩng tyme draweth towarde heate, the more the vryne gethereth hygh colour, departyng frõ pale and flaxen, toward palew & light safferne: & the inequalyte of substaũce chaungeth into a dewe equalytie accordyng to nature, and the grounde doth waxe thynner, & the quantytie is more in respecte to that is dronke: so that about the myddest of the spring they retourne to a meane. In the beginnyng of summer the colour appereth palew

Summer

and lyght saffren, and the substaunce meane, the ground whyte, dewly knyt & stable, but yet thynner then a meane grounde. And the more that the sũmer procedeth and draweth to the highest, the lesser is the quantytie of vryne in comparysõ to the drynke, & the groũd chaũgeth from his naturall whytenes to a palysh colour, & is moch lesser and thynner. And this thynnes glystereth with all and enclyneth toward golden

Heruest

and saffren coloure.   When Heruest cummeth, then the coloures rrtourne
to a

OF VRINE. 21.

to a menes agayne: but the thynnesse and bȝightnesse remayneth styll, the grounde alſo is ſtyll obſcure and lytle, but yet it is white, deuly knyt & ſtable. And as herueſt goeth foȝward, ſo the vȝine returneth to a meane in all thinges. In the myddle of wynter & there about, the vȝine kepeth dew quantitie, but the colour enclineth toward white and the ground is ouer great, but in al other pointes it is mene. And as wynter goeth on, the ſubſtaunce of vȝyne appereth dyuerſe, & the colour whyte, the quantytie greater in reſpect to the dȝinke, and the contentes greater and vnconcocte, but toward the ſpȝynge tyme they retourne towarde a meane, as I haue befoȝe ſayd. Yet beſyde theſe alſo dyuerſytie of coūtreyes cauſeth dyuerſytie of vȝyne, euen by the ſame reaſons as doth the tymes of the yere. Foȝ coūtreyes that be temperate exactly, make vȝine lyke vnto yͤ ſpȝing tyme. And thoſe countreyes that be hotte and dȝye make vȝyne lyke vnto ſummer. And contrary wayes colde & moyſt alter water as dothe wynter.

Wynter

Countreys

Countreys

D.v. But

THE IVDICIALL

Meates drynkes & medicynes.

But countreyes that are drye and distempered betwene heate & colde, make vryne lyke heruest. Also meates and drynkes and order of dyete causeth vryne to alter, & medicynes also, as not only experyēce teacheth, but also Hippocrates wytnesseth in the .vj. boke of his Epidemys (or rainyng sicknesses) in the .v. parte & the .rv. sentence: as for example. Those meates that are lyght of concoction and good in substaunce, cause good and temperate vryne with pure contentes: but contrary meates cause discoloured vryne and thynne, with straunge contentes.

Meates that wyll not concoct, make lesser contentes, & dyuerse in substaūce. Euyll meates cause greater contentes and in nothyng duly formed. And as the qualitie of meates doth alter vrine, so dothe the quātitie also. For if a man haue eaten moche, & not concocted it, his vryne shalbe thynne & whyte, and sumtyme without grounde. But if this crudyte (or rawnesse in stomake) contynew long, the vryne wyll be cum dyuerse in substaunce, and in contentes.

Also

OF VRINE. 22.

Also wyne dronke abundautly, causeth alteration in vrpne. But now contrary wayes, if a man do fast long, his vrine wyll appere fyrie and saffren coloured and thynne, with lesser ground. But if a man suffer famyn & doo not nourysh, his water shalbe thynne & whyte with a certeyn glysteryng, & without grouũ. More ouer exercyce and rest chaungeth *Labour* vrpne: for thorow excessyue labour, the vrpne chaungeth from lyght saffren, & at lengthe becummeth saffren coloured with lytle grounde, thynne, & hygher coloured then it shuld be. And sumtime there fleeteth on the toppe a certeyne fattynes, specially after ouer moch wetynesse. But idlenesse & rest dothe con- *Reste* trary wayes cause whyte vrpne, with greater and grosser grounde. Further- *Sleepe* more, sleepe, and watchyng, if they ex- *Watchyng* cede measure, they alter vrpne: but there is difference betwene bothe sleepe and watchyng cummyng of sycknesse, & them bothe when they be taken wyllyngly in health. For if that sycknesse cause ouer moche sleepe, then is the vrpne whytysh, whith substaũce other ful
      ly thyck

THE IVDICIAL

ly thycke, or but party thynne, and the contentes many and vndygest. But if that soche sleepe cum naturally, the vryne is not so whyte, but rather flaxen, and the substaunce meane, with greater and well concocte contentes. And lyke wayes they that haue watched purposedly & not by reason of sycknesse, their vrine is but lytle chaũged. But if they watche for any syckly cause, their vryne wyl chaũge but lytle at the beginnyng: but with contynuaunce the contentes wyll be dysparsed, & at last cleane wasted, & the substaunce of the vryne waxeth thynner & thynner by lytle & lytle, & the colour enclineth other to whyte and watery: other to golden, saffren, oylye, or blacke, accordĩg as the cause is, that maketh it so to chaunge. Of alteration by complexiõ, I wyll wryte in the next chappter. Now haue you herde as touchyng alteration of uryne in helth, accordyng to dyuersytie of ages bothe in men and women, tymes of the yere, countreys, meates & drynkes, laboure, rest, sleepe & watche: so that you must haue regarde to these, in al iudgemetes

bothe

OF VRINE. 23.

bothe in health and in sicknesse. For if these be nott dilygently marked, they may cause great error as you may well consyder. Fyrst therfore in euery vrpne you must cõsidre whether it be a mãns or a womannes, and what age he or she is of: then what tyme of the yere it is, and what countrey, what meates and drynkes the person vsed: & lyke wayes of labor & rest, sleepe and watche: and then must you consydre how euery one of these dothe alter vrpne: so that if the alteryng of them from that helthful v=ryne (wherof I spake in the beginning of this chapiter) be but soche as one of those foresayd thinges wold cause, then may it not be iudged to cum of any dis=ease, as for example: Hygh coloured water in somer (so that it passe not saf=ferne coloure) or whyte coloured water in wynter, shulde rather be rekoned to cum of the time of the yere, then of any sycknesse: & lyke wayes of other thĩges.

What be the generall qualyties that alter the partes of Uryne.
The .vii. Chapiter.

Before

THE IVDICIALL

Efore I intreate of the fygnifycation of the partes of vrpne, I thynke it good to inſtructe you of the generall qualyties, which cauſe all alterations in vrpne: whereby you ſhall perceyue not onely what euery vrpne doth betoken (as I ſhall a non ſet furth) but alſo if you marke well this chapiter, you ſhall ſee the cauſe why euery vrpne dothe ſo ſygnify.

You ſhall vnderſtand therfore that there be .iiij. cheefe and only qualyties wherof all thynges that ar both in the ſee & earth are made: as man & beaſt: fyſh & foule: trees, herbes, ſtones and metals. Theſe .iiij. qualyties ar heate, colde, moyſtneſſe and dryneſſe: & theſe iiij. contynuyng duly tempered (as nature ordered them fyrſt in euery pfyte body) be the cauſe of contynual helth. But if they be altered wronglp, then doo they cauſe dyſeaſes dyuerſely, accordyng to the dyuerſytie of the alterations. And as they doo cauſe dyſeaſes, ſo they chauge þ colour, ſubſtauce, and other partes of the vrpne, wherby we may coniecture the cauſe of the diſ=

eaſe

OF VRINE 24.

eafe : and fo confequently the dyfeafe it felfe, though fumtyme it declareth the difeafe it felf, & not the caufe therof

But now to come to the mater meteſt for this tyme, you ſhal marke, that ij. of thefe .iiij. qualities ar named paſſyue, and they caufe but ſmall alteration in comparyſon. The other .ij. are called actyue, and they caufe great alteratiõ. The actyue qualyties ar heate and colde, & the paſſyue qualyties are dryneſſe & moyſtneſſe. When moyſtnes therfore exceedeth alone, it dulleth the naturall colour of vryne, thycketh and engroſſeth the ſubſtaunce and encreaſeth the quãtytie. And as the ouer parte of it aboue waxeth rough & troubled, ſo the grounde encreſeth & contynueth raw & vnconcocte. But dryneſſe dothe dyminyſh the quantytie of vryne and alſo the contentes: It maketh it thynne in ſubſtaũce, cleare and bryght, and cauſeth meane coloure, & the grounde appereth groſſer.

Lyke waies heate, if it excede meaſure but lytle, it maketh palew & lyght ſaffern colour in the vryne. But if heat excyde

Moyſtneſſe

Dryneſſe

Heate

THE IVDICIAL

excyde greatly, it canseth golden and safferne colour, with meane substaũce, and a lytle bryghtnesse: the grounde is meane in respecte to the quãtytie of v=ryne, but it declyneth from the dew whytenesse toward safferne coloure.

Colde

But colde on the other syde maketh vryne tourne to whyte coloure, and chaũgeth the substaunce frõ a meane. And if the colde increase, the vryne wyl alter from meane substaũce, & therfore consequently wyll be other thynne, o=ther grosse. If it be thynne or vnpure the grounde shall be other obscure and lytle, other moche, & that dyuerse and vncõcocte. And this is the worrking of these .iiij. qualyties when they excyde alone. But and if .ij. of them excyde together, there may result of that sort iiij. other dystemperaunces: as hotte and drye, hotte and moyst, colde & dry, and colde and moyst. Now what alte=rations these & euery one of them doth cause in vryne, you may easely coniec=ture, if you keepe in mynd that, that I saide of the .iiij. symple qualyties: and so adde together the alterations. And this

Compound distempe= ratures of qualytyes

OF VRINE. 25.

this must you remēber therewith, that where they both agre in any alteratiō they cause that alteratiō to be the greter: and where they be contrary, they cause the alteration to be nearer to a meane: howe be it sumwhat to helpe you, take this brefe declaration. As a temperate man doth make that parfecte vrpne wrytten of before, so the vrpne of a sanguyne man (which is hot and moyst) shall be yelow, or lyght safferne coloured, by the reasō of ẏ heat, and sumwhat grosse, by the reason of the moysture. In a coloricke man (beyng hotte and dry) the vrpne shall be in coloure as in a sanguyne man, but in substaūce thynne, by reason of the drynesse. The vrpne of a melancolye man (whose nature is colde and drye) shall be whyte thorough the colde, and cleare, for the drynesse. The phlegmatycke man (which is colde and moyst) maketh vrpne whyte thorough colde, and thyck by the moysture. For as heat and colde altereth the coloures, so drynesse and moysture chaungeth the substaunce. Now if you haue remēbred

C.j.   all

THE IVDICIAL

all that I haue wrytten before, then shal you be the meeter, and better able a great deale to perceyue the reasons oʒ the tokens which vryne doth geue. And so shal your knoulege be the moʒe certeyn, if you know not only the thig but also the cause of it. Now therfore wyll I wryte of the sygnifycations of the partes of vryne partyculerly, that you may perceyue that fyrst and cheife commodytie of vryne which it worketh for mannes health.

The sygnifycations of the partes of vryne partyculerly   The, viii. Chapiter.

I Told you in the .vj. chapiter of this boke, what vryne was most parfect sownde, and healthfull of all other: And I sayde that it was the rule and tryall to exampn all other vrynes by: so that the nearer that any vryne were vnto it, the better it were: and the further that it declyneth fro it, the worse it is. This (I sayde) shulde be as a generall rule: which thyng to be trew in healthfull men, you may perceyue by that I haue written all redy. And that it is

OF VRINE. 26.

it is also trew in sycke men, Hyppocrates wytnesseth, sayeng: That vryne is best, whose ground is whyte, duly knyt and stable, all the tyme the syckenesse preuayleth. But Galen, to supply that that is vnderstand in this sayeng, and so to make it parfecte, addeth thereto: That it must be of colour partye golden or palew, and of a meane substaũce betwene thycke and thynne. And also in these thynges is requyred stablenes, to make it a parfecte vryne: for that that is vnstable in any parte, in that it is not parfecte. Here were a place to speke of the difference of this chaungeablenesse or vnstablenesse: for there is one sorte called ordynary, and a nother called vnordynary / and of both these are there dyuerse dyfferences. But bycause they depend of an exacter iudgement then vnlerned me can wel atteyn vnto, I ouer passe them for this tyme, and wyll declare the other dyfferences of vryne, whereby it altereth frõ this meane vrine, in al partes particulerly. And fyrst I wyl begynne with the substaunce of vryne, the which (as I sayd before) *Substaũce*

E.ij.

THE IVDICIAL

Meane

beforꝭ) is of iij. kyndes, thyck, thynne and meane. A meane vryne is that, that is in the myddle betweene extreme thycke, and extreme thynne. And as it is meane betwene them in substaũce, so is it meane in sygnifycation / for it doth betokẽ (of it selfe) only good temperaunce & health. But the other .ij. be token distẽperaunce & defaulte of concoction, & that dyuersly, accordyng to the diuersytie of the causes of them, as you shal now cõsequẽtly heare. Fyrst, to speke of thynne vryne, other it doth styl so contynew thynne, as it was fyrst made, other elles it dothe shortly waxe thycke and troubled. That that doth contynew styll thynne, doth betoken lacke of concoction, & so doth the other also: but yet this that cõtinueth thinne betokeneth more lacke of concoction: for it betokeneth that nature hath not yet begon to concocte. And therfore is that water, a sygne of extreme crudytie or rawnesse in nature. But that that waxeth thycke, after it begynneth to coole, though it betoken lacke of concoction, yet doth it declare that nature

Thynne vryne

hath

OF VRINE 27.

hathe begon to concocte all redye, not withstandyng it is an euyll vryne, for it signifieth that nature hath nede, not only of great streugth to performe that concoction which she hath begon, but also that there is requyred long tyme to the performaunce of the same. For the which cause Galen calleth this, of all vrynes the worst. This haue you herde touchyng crudytie and concoctiõ what thynne vryne doth sygnifye, so that all thynne vrine betokeneth cru= dytte. And besyde that, it doth further betoken (as wytnesseth Hippocrates) getheringes or apostumations in the nether partes of the body, namely, if it contynew so very longe, and the pa= cyent escape death. Further more, if soch thynne vrine haue with it a lyght whytenesse, it is a very euyll sygne. For if it be in a burnyng Ague, it is a token of frensycknesse. But if the pacyent be frensycke all redy, and the vryne dothe so continew, it doth most commynly be token death. And if he escape death (the whiche is seldome sene) then shall he be longe sycke, and escape hardly.

Thynne & whyte

E.iij. Thynne

THE IVDICIALL

Thynne vryne also betokeneth dyuerse other thynges: as the stoppyng of the raynes, and of the water vaynes. And lyke wayes, if a man haue had moche bledyng, or laxe, or pyssyng, his vryne wyll be whyte and thynne, and almost without ground. Lyke maner, in olde age, and longe weakenesse of sycknes. Also in yonge chyldren, if it contynew longe, it is a deadly sygne. Yet thyn vrine doth sumtime betoken eande of sycknes and recouery of health: as in Agues (namely cotidianes) if at the beginnyng of them and so after, the v=ryne dyd appere thycke and troubled / especially if the colour ameð therwith,

Thyn and flaxen

And if it be thynne in substaūce, and of flaxen colour, then is it better then thynne and whyte: for bycause the co=lour is better though the substaūce be all one / so that though it betoken sum wekenesse and lacke of concoction, yet not so moch as dothe the other, for the colour is meanely concocte: that is to say, natural heate is menely creseð.

Thyn and golden.

But if it be thynne & golden, it is yet more better then thynne and flaxen:

for

OF VRINE 28.

for the colour is moꝛe exacte / and this betokeneth concoctiõ halfe complete: for that that is lacked in substaunce, it hath in colour. After this is there thynne & safferne coloured, which betokeneth fyꝛst, lacke of concoction, and besyde that, defaulte of noꝛyshment / as in a yong man that fasteth longe. And sumtyme it betokeneth that excesse of heate in the inner partes of the body, dothe cause colerycke humours to abounde, as in the feuer tertian. Besyde all this, it betokeneth thought, carefulnesse, and watchyng, and also ouer muche labour, and takyng of heate in the sonne. And this haue you herde the sygnifycations of thynne vꝛyne, bothe a lone, & also with soch coloures as it can be cowpyllyd. Now shall you heare what thycke vꝛine doth betoken bothe alone, & olso with soche dyuerse coloures, as it may be cowpyllyd.

 Thycke vꝛyne which is so (I meane when it is fyꝛst made) other it dothe continew styll thycke, other els it doth settle, and waxe cleare. If it contynew styll thycke, it betokeneth that that disturbaūce

Thyn and safferne

Thycke

C.iiij.

THE IVDICIAL

turbaunce, which was in the blood, that is to say, the rage of sycknes, doth styll contynew strongly: and that naturall strength is but weake. this vryn is not so good as that which doth settell, and waxe cleare, for that doth betoken, that the dysease shall shortly be ouercum: how be it there remayneth yet sumwhat of that dystemperate trobell in the blood. Yet nature hath the ouer hand, and expelleth the mater of the greefe, and therfore is soch a vryn called good. but yet it betokeneth sum lacke of concoctiõ, though not so moch as that which contynueth troubled & thycke styll. Also thycke vryne (if it be excedyng thycke) doth betoken death, as Hippocrates sayth. And the vryne that is thycke and troubled, lyke beastes vryne, doth betoken head ache, other present all redy, or shortly after to cum. If thycke vryne appere in an ague, where thynne vryne went before, it betokeneth that the sycknesse wyll abate streyght wayes, for it declareth that nature hath ouercum the mater of the sycknesse: but if it appere thicke
at the

OF VRINE. 29.

at the begynnyng of the Ague, & doo not waxe thynne in pcesse of tyme, it betokeneth plenty of mater, & wekenes of nature, so that there is feare, lest nature shalbe ouercũ, except ỹ colour do amende. Thycke vryne also betokeneth openness of the water pypes & reynes. And if it be thycke and whyte, it betokeneth great plenty of raw humours, & sũdry kyndes of flewme to be gethered in the body, & betokeneth also (namely if it be moche) that those getherynges, which mought be loked for in fore Agues, shall not ensew: for the mater which shuld cause them, departeth out by vryne: but the whyteness of this vryne is bryght as snowe. For if it be sumwhat darkerlyke ỹ whyteness of mylke, it is a token of the stone, other in the bledder or reynes, namely if soch vrine chaunce in the ende & a mending of sickenes: but yf ỹ color of it be grey, it betokenith not only plẽty of mater in the body, but also that the hole body is possessed with a daũgerous syckenes. whereof oftẽ tymes it chaũceth ỹ paciẽt to breke out w blisters & hete in his skyn.

Thycke & whyte

Grey

E.v.

THE IVDICIALL

*Thycke &
Claret*

Nexte after this foloweth thycke & cla red colour (for flaxen, yellow, nor saf= ferne colour doth not agree with thyck vryne) and it doth sygnify that the dis= ease shall contynew longe, specyally if the grounde of it be also of claret colour. But yet is this disease without peryll of death.

*Thycke &
redd*

Thycke vryne, if it be red coloured, doth betoken abundaunce of blood, as is sene in contynuall Agues, and in all peryllous Agues, as wytnes= seth Theophilus. If this water cum by lytle and lytle, it is an euyll token / for it doth alwayes declare daunger. And if that sorte of vryne (in soche A= gues) doo waxe troubled, so that there cum with it defenes of hearyng, and ache of the headd, with payne in the necke and in the sydes of the belly, it betokeneth that the pacyent shall haue the Fallyng euyll within a seuenyght.

*Thycke ād
Crymsen*

And if a thycke vryne haue a crymsen colour, if it be inburnyng Agues, and the pacyent then haue the hed ache, it betokeneth that a cheife crytycall sygne

*Thycke ād
blew*

other is then present, or elles nygh at hande. But if the vryne be thycke & blew

OF VRINE.   30.

blew coloured, it sygnifyeth dyuersely as the persones are that made it. For in them that are in way of recouery, it betokeneth that they shall escape their greife. It sygnifyeth also payne in the water pipes, or els that the party hath rūne moche. And if it appere soche in olde men, and that contynew longe, it declareth not onely that the bladder is infected with euyll humours / but commenly also that he shal be ryd of them. But if it cum after the greife of the stone, it declareth that, that greife shall be turned into ỹ strangury. Thycke vryne and greene, namely in Agues, is a token of the yellow Jawnders, other present or redy to cum. Thycke vrine & asshe coloured, if it appere in Agues and do not settle, it is a sygne of madnesse. But in the burnyng Ague, it betokeneth that the Strãgury wyll cum shortly. But if blacke coloure appere in thicke vryne, it betokeneth somtyme well, as in the ende of the Feuer quarten, and of melancolyke madnesse / for it betokeneth that the melãcolyke mater, which caused the dyseases, dothe avoyde

Thycke ãd greene

Thycke ãd aſh colored

Thycke ãd blacke

THE IVDICIAL

voyde out. But sumtymes it is an euyl token, for it sygnifyeth that either the blood is burned through excedīg heat, or els that natural heate is clene quēched through dedly colde, & therfore is it cōmenly called a dedly signe, namely in sharpe Agues, if it haue an euyll sauour. And so meneth Galen, when he saith that he markyd: the thicker that a blacke water is, the worse it is: and more ouer: that he neuer saw any escape, which made soch vryne. And thus haue you herde of the significations of thynne & thycke vryne, with soch colours as may be couppylled therwith.

Now wyll I wrytte a lytle of the coloures alone, & of soch tokens as cum chefely of them, rather then of the substaūce or any other parte of the vrine.

Coloures of vryne

The colours of vryn declare cōmenly, how heate and colde do reygne in the body: so that the whyter the vryne is, the greater is the colde, and naturall heate the lesse: & the hygher coloured that the vryn is, ẙ greater is the hete. But to speke ptyculerly, that you may

Whyte

parceyue it the better. If the vryne be
whyte

OF VRINE. 31.

whyte, it is a sygne that cōcoction fay= leth quyte, & the lyghter coloured, the worse. Pale colour is beter sumwhat, though it also declare lacke of natural heate & strenght. And flaxen coloure, though it betoken beginnyng of con= coction, yet is it not parfecte: how be it it may be wel taken, if all other signes be good. Palew and lyght safferne (as you haue herde before) are the best co= loures, & most temperate, which betokē exact concoction. But golden & saffrē colour declare excesse of heate. Claret is nexte, & then red, after it crymsen, & then purple, then greene, & last of them is oyly vzyne: which as they go in oz= der, so thei declare greater and greater heate with increase, not onely of the qualytie, but also of mater conteinyng the same. But now of the other syde: blew vzyne, & asshe colour, are tokens of excessyue colde, sumtyme w̄ mater, & sumtime w̄out: & so lyke ways of black vzyne, how be it, it cūmeth sumtyme of excesse of hete. but how you may know the differences both of it, and all the other, now wyll I shew in ozder, with the rest of their sygnifycations.

Pale

Flaxen

Palew Lyght saf= ferne

Golden Safferne Claret Red Crymsen Purple Greene Oylye

Blew Ash colour

THE IVDICIALL

Whyt

Whyte vryne, if it cum in great quan‐
tytie in a hole mã, it betokeneth moche
drinkyng of thynne wyne. But if it be
meane in quantytie, with a due groũd,
it declareth colde dystemperaũce of the
lyuer. The vryne doth appere whyte,
with a dyfforme and vnconcocted
ground, in them that haue the dropsy.
But in olde mẽ, whyte vryne is no gret
euyll sygne, as you may parceyue by
that I sayd before of Ages, how they
alter vryne. But in yong men, & soche
as ar of freshest age, it is a worse sygne
and specially if it haue other no con‐
tentes, other els euyll contentes. And
if vryne contynew long tyme whyte,
without chaungeyng, it betokeneth
paynful beatyng of the head, daselling
of the eyes, and gyddynesse, & also the
fallyng euyll, lothsumnesse of good
meates, and lustyng sumtyme after e‐
uyll meates, greedy hunger, payne in
the lymmes, and paynfull mouyng of
the sennowes, and dyuerse greefes of
the head and raynes / and also payne
in the fundement, and great weakenes
by syckenesse : for all these do follow
con‐

OF VRINE 34.

contynuall lacke of concoction, other colde, other stoppyng of the vaynes & isshewes, other transposyng of the humours. But y̌ differences of these can not easely be knowen of euery mā / but soche as are lerned may gether certein dystinctions of them by the accydētes which follow dyseases. Darke whyte coloures, as mylke whyte, whyte lyke horne, and grey: If they appere in the begynnyng of Agues & in the increase of them, they do betoken moch payn. But in the decrease of agues, they declare health, specially if it cum plentyfully. Pale vryne and flaxen doo not lyghtly appere in Agues, excepte they be easy Agues, & shorte as those which contynew but one daye: but if that it do follow after burnyng Agues, it declareth that they be fully dyssolued. As for palew and lyght safferne, they are (as I sayde before) the best & most parfecte colours, namely in yong men and fresh youth. But in olde men, women and chyldren (whose vryne, as I haue sayde, declyneth toward whyte & pale) it doth betoken that their body is to hotte

mylk whyt
horne whyt
Grey.

Pale. flaxen

Palew
safern

TEE IVDICIAL

to hotte, other by reason of their dyete or els of their excersyce. But in as moch as it is but meane excesse, it declareth but small greife. Golden and safferne coloured vryne, if it be other sumwhat thynne, or very thycke, other it hath no grounde, or elles very few & darke contentes. But in this they dyffer, that golden vryn declareth excesse of heate and mater also, by reason of meates, sharpe medicynes, chafyng of the blood thorow anger, heate of the bowels, or els heate of the tyme of the yere. But safferne colour appereth rather with defaulte of mater, thorough sum affection of the mynde, watchyng, heate of the sonne, laboure, & soche lyke thiges, which encrease thynne & yellow choler, and dimynysh naturall heate, so that the cause of this colour is, choler it selfe increased other in quantytie, or els in qualytie. But in olde men, & women, & soche other, there is sum greater cause that occasyoneth it, for it sygnifyeth an Ague cummyng of saffernly choler, dysperfed thorough the hole body : After which there followeth commenly, gyddynesse,

Golden Safferne Colour

OF VRINE. 33.

dynes, hed ache, bitternes of the mouth
lothsumnes of meate, thurstines. Also
in yong men, soch vrine is caused
thorough moch exercyse, &
vse of hotte meates.

Of claret and redde Vryne.

Claret and redd vrine is coloured other of the myxture of red choler, or els of the corruption of blood: soch vrine often tymes goeth before Agues. For whē the blood doth so abound that it can not be duly laboured, nor can take no ayer, there is engendred a certen corruption, which as it is red of colour it selfe, so it causeth the vryne to be red in colour, if it be moch, els it maketh onley claret colour. But if it be exacte red, lyke grayne, it betoketh that blood yshoweth into it out of sum vaynes nygh to the raynes, which other are broken, or other wayes opened. But how it may be knowen from whence it cummeth & how, there ar may meanes to serche: but bicause they ar not lyght to perceyue, I wyl reserue them for phyficions that are learned. This colour

F.j.   of it

THE IVDICIAL,

of it felfe is no great euyll fygne, namely in yong men: for it betokeneth exceffe of blood, whiche may well be borne of them. But in olde men it is a very euyll fygne / for it betokeneth other long fyckeneffe, or els death: fyth nature is fo weke, that it can not kepe in hyr naturall humour. And if that redd coloure cum of redd choler, as it doth in yong men for the moft parte, & not of blood (which thynge a lernyd Phyficion may coniecture partely by the former dyete, & other fygnes mo) the accydentes fhal be the moare troubeloufe: how be it yet not fo euyll, as when it cummeth of faferen or golden choler: for this caufeth greter thurft & more troubeloufe flepe, then the other.

Of Crymfen colour

Crymfen coloure is a token that the good humoures of the body ar burned, & turned vnto red or black choler, which caufe worfe grefes thẽ ỹ other: howbeit if it haue a good ground, the grefe is the moare moderate. But if it haue other no coutentes for a fpace,
or els

OF VRINE. 34

oꝛ els euyll contentes, and the vꝛyne appere lyke a thycke myſte, but ſum=what glyſterynge lyght, it is a ſygne that nature nedeth moch ſtrengthe to recouer her ſelfe to her owne ſtate. Notwithſtandyng ſoch vꝛyne is cau=ſed ſumtymes in hole folke, by reaſon of moch labour and longe iourneyng, & then it hath ſum good ſygnes there=with. But in them that haue a ſharpe Ague, ſoch crymſen coloure of vꝛyne doth betokẽ, that coꝛrupte blood doth abounde, and that it doth putrify, and turne into choler. And commynly thei that make ſoch vꝛyne, do thyꝛſt moch and are dꝛye in their mouth, and are troubyllyd in their ſlepe, & fele ſharpe Agues, and ar halfe dyſtracte, and fele payne of the lyuer, with coughyng. houbeit, yet theſe ſignes mai be ſutims as well good as bad, accoꝛding as the colours do chaũge, to better oꝛ woꝛſe.

Of Purple colour.

Purple coloure declareth nede of moche ſtrengthe befoꝛe it can be al=tered to a good vꝛyne.

F.ij. This

THE IVDICIAL

This vrin is a sygne of burned choler. And if it do contynew very long, it is a token of the yellow Jaunders, with abundaunce of grosse & corrupte choler, gathered in the lyuer. And at the beginning there goeth with it sum spices and grudgynges of the Ague, with a lytle thurstynesse: but vnlesse there be discretiō vsed in ye dyete of soch a paciēt it may turne to a moch worse disease.

Of greene Vrines

Grene coloure is an euyll & a daungerous token, for it nedeth not only long tyme, but also continual strength, to brynge it a gayne too a good trade. The hygher that this coloure is, the more it declareth that choler excedeth the other humoures: which if it be any more burned, wyll cause blacke vryne, of which I wyll a none speake. but if grene colour cum of wasting of the fat, then is it sumwhat lyke to oyly colour or popynjay grene: but if it cum of a bundaunce of purpellysh choler, and thorough increase of his qualytie, then doth the coloure inclyne more toward blacke,

OF VRINE 35.

blacke, & glyſterith with ſhadowy grene drawyng very nygh vnto blacke.

After grene choler followeth madnes, parbrakyng and auoidyng of choler, ſumtymes alone, & ſumtimes with matter or els burned: and alſo contynuall thurſtyneſſe and burnyng, heate of the tong, ſtrayghtneſſe about the ſtomake, and lyke other thynges. But if the pacyent contynew ſtrong, and the coloure of the vryne do waxe lyghter, there is good hope, els there is great feare, leſt of the dryneſſe and burnyng there doo folow contractiõ of the ſenowes, which wyll kyll the pacyent.

Of oyly vryne or Popyngey greene

Oyly vryne is of .iij. ſortes, as I ſeyd in the .v. chapiter. that is light oyly, ſtarke oylye and darke oylye.

Oylye vrynes ar a token of vnnaturall heate, & the hygher that the colour is, the greater is the heate. And alſo they betoken moltyng of the fatte within a man, for of it are they ſo coloured. But at the beginnyng, when there is lyttle fatte molted, the vryne is lyght oylye,

F.iij.   For

THE IVDICIAL

For if it loke starke oylye, then it sygnifieth that the disease increaseth. But if it cum ones to darke oily, then is the dysease sore increased. Hippocrates in the .vij. boke of his Aphorismys speking of fatnes in vrine, sayth thus: Who so maketh vrine with a fatye flottes cummyng moch and fast, they haue sharpe paynes in the raynes. Which sentence though it might seme more to appertayne to the contentes then to the colour, yet doth not only Galen, but also Aëti' Actuari', & also an other grecyã (whose name I know not) expoũd it amongest coloures: & by it declare the dyfference, to know whether that waste or moltyng of fatte be in the raines self, or in other partes of the body. For if it cum fast together, (as Hyppocrates saith) then cũmeth it from the raynes self, & betokeneth the wastyngg to be in them. But if it cum softly & increse bi litle & litle, then doth it declare that yͤ hole body is ouercum w̃ vnnatural hete, & that yͤ fat of it doth wast: & doth betokẽ (as Act. witnesseth) a wastyng Ague, cõsumyng the body.

Of

OF VRINE   36.

Of Blew vryne, Aſhcolour and Blacke.

BLew colour, Aſhecoloure & Blacke, do dyffer only in lyghtneſſe & darkeneſſe. For aſhecoloure is darker then blew : & blacke is darker then any of them both. Blew colour ſumtyme cummeth of moderate melancholy, & then is the vzyne ſumwhat thynne in ſubſtaunce : & ſumtyme it cũmeth of great colde, & then is it thicke in ſubſtaunce. And ſumtyme it is a token of moztifyeng of ſum parte. Yea, and ſumtyme euen of hole nature : namely, if the colour chaunge to woꝛſe & woꝛſe, & there went befoꝛe no token of concoction.

Aſhecoloured vzyne cũmeth of lyke cauſes & betokeneth lyke thĩges. how beit it is ſo coloured many tymes, whẽ the partye that made it, hath ben ſoꝛe betẽ & bꝛuſed. But in this you nede not ẙ helpe of vꝛin, foꝛ you mai ſe ẙ waltes and tokens of the ſtrypes in his body.

Uryn which is extreme blacke, ſumtyme betokeneth extreme heate, & ſum tyme extreme colde : the whiche both you may diſtynctely dyſcerne, if you doo obſerue oꝛder of alteration in the colours of the vzyne that the pacyent

THE IVDICIALL

made last before. For if his vrpne before were greene, or lyke therto, then doth the blacke vrpne which followeth it, betoken extreme heate. But if it were last before blew or asshecoloured, then doth it sygnifye extreme colde. This blacke colour, though it be commenly an euyll and deadly sygne (as I sayde before, speakyng of thycke vrpne and blacke) yet sumtyme it is a good token.

For in all dyseases lyghtly that cum of melãcholy mater, it betokeneth that the mater doth auoyde, and so the syckenesse to ende. And soch vrine doth appere many tymes, after purgations or other meates & drikes which purge the splene: namely if a man do laboure vpon them, and was before dysased of the splene. how be it, sumtyme meates and drinkes of lyke colour, cause black vrpne, as Galene wytnesseth, namely after darke red wyne and Allegaunte. But in moderate Agues, if soch blacke vrpne do appere, it is a token of death, excepte it be on sum cryptcall dayes. And lyke ways in sharpe Agues, especially if the sauour be strong & stynkig:
vnlesse

OF VRINE. 39

vnles it cum of sum grefe of y̆ bladder. Let this suffyce for this tyme, as tou=chyng colours. Now for the quantitie of vryn, as whē it is mene, it is a good token: so when it is other to moch o=ther to lytle, it is an euyll sygne, except it cum of sum soch cause, as I shewed before, that altereth vrpne in a health=full man. As fyrst excessyue quantite of vrpne, cummeth of moch drinkyng of thinne wyne, as renysh wyne, & soch lyke. But that shall you thus knowe: for the colour wyll be whytelye, & the substaunce thynner then a meane, the contentes also wyll be dyuerse, & not duly knytte. Lykewyse if there be a=bundaunce of raw humoures in a mā vnconcocted, & yet nature perseueryng strong, then is there great quantytie of vrpne, and sumwhat thynne of sub=staūce, but not so whyte as that other, & the contentes of this are better. Also (as Hippocrates sayth), moche vrpne made in the nyght, is a token of small sege: so that if any impedyment lett naturall sege, then wyll the quantytie of vrpne be the greater. But in this,

F.v. as

Quantytie,

Moch in a hole bodye

4. Aphor. 3

THE IVDICIAL

as the colour is meane, so is the groūd both greater & grosser. Yet in helthful folke may the vryn, by another menys also, be greter thē a meane: & that may be by medicyns which prouoke vryne. But then is the coloure more naturall then the last þ I spoke of, & the groūde is thynner of substaunce: so that it is darke & scarsely sene, & then is there a certayne glysterpng in the vrpne selfe.

Lytle vryne in a hole bo dye.

Now cōtrary ways, & of cōtrary cau=ses cūmeth small quantytie of vrpn. For it cūmeth sūtyme of lacke of drinke or drye meates, & then is the colour lyght safren, w̄ a smal groūd, but yet sūthing grosse. Also both meates & medicyns þ ar clāmy, & apte to stop þ water pipes, do cause lytle vrin, but then is þ groūd also litle & thynne. Besides these, moch sege causeth vrpn to be lesser: for if the one excremētes be greater then nature wold, the other must nedes be lesse, if the bodye be helthful. In this vrpn, as you may partely know þ cause of it by the knowledge of the excessyue sege, so wyll the vrpn selfe be thynner, and the ground very darke, thynne, & not duly
knyt.

OF VRINE. 29.

knyt. And this many wayes may this alteration appere in a helthfull body.

Now in a sycke persone moch vryne other betokeneth the dropsy : & then is it lyke water with a rawe and dyuerse grounde. Other els if it be whyte, thyn, & without grounde, then doth it betokẽ the pyssyng euyll. And this vryne (as wytnesseth Galen in his fyrst boke of iudicialles) is the worst of any other of lyke sorte (I meane, whiche declare lacke of concoction) for it declareth the decay, yea I may say, the vtter extinc=tiõ of two naturall powres, that is the retentyue power, & the alteratyue po=wer alsō. Moch vryn, in colour fyrie, and lyght safren, or of any lyke colour, is to be feared : namely, if it be com=pelyd with euyll contentes. But if it be of crymsen or purple colour, and so procede, especyally if no concoction went before it, then doth it enclyne to euyll, and betokeneth a certayne mor=tyfyeng, and wastyng of the hole com=posycion of the body. But if moche vryne cum in an Ague, namely to=warde the ende, and that there went
before

Moche v= ryne in a sycke body

Diabete.

THE IVDICIALL

before it lytle vryne, thycke & cruddy, then is that a good toke̅, as witnesseth Hippocrates, for it betokeneth the Ague to be at an ende. and this vryne wyl be whyte and thynne moderately, and wyll haue a meane grounde.

4. Apho. 69

Now lytle quantytie of vryne, with a grosse grounde, vnduly knyt and vnconcocte, is an euyll token, for it betokeneth the wekenes of the alteratyue power, which is not able to extenuate, concocte, nother alter the mater, and therfore doth it with moch diffycultie passe forth in soch grossenes. How be it if there follow after it a more thynner vryne, with the ground well & duly knyt, & stable, then is it without feare. For this later vryne (as you herde before) is a token that the cause of the other is ouercum and vainquyshed. This lytle quantytie of vryne cu̅meth sumtyme in vehement Agues, & then is the vyolent heate cause there of. Sumtime also it cummeth of the stoppyng of the water pypes, nott onely thorough clammy meates & drynkes, but also of sum dysease or greefe in the̅.

Lytle vryne in a sycke body

And

OF VRINE 39

And this now shal suffyce for an introduction, as touchyng the substaunce, coloures, and quantytie of vryne.

It followeth nexte, to speake of the contentes, whiche so greatly helpe too the ryght iudgement of vryne, that Hippocrates (in his seconde booke of Prognostications) doth by them only, yea, and that by one of them (I meane the ground) pronounce the iudgement of a parfecte vryne: sayeng, that that is the best vryne, which hath his sedyment or grounde, whyte, duly knyt, & stable, & that contynually all the tyme of the syckenesse. Now seyng this great clerke and father of Physicke, doth thus esteme the grounde. it shall not seme vnmeete, that I orderly doo wryte breefely of those principall thinges that be too be consydered as touchyng the contentes, and fyrst of all of the grounde, which hath alteration (as you haue herde) both in substaūce, coloure & quantytie. But now as touchyng the substaunce, then is it onely meane, when the thyrd concoction in the veynes is parfecte. For the ground is the

Contentes.

Sedyment

TEE IVDICIAL

is the excrement (as you myght say) of that thyrde concoction. And is lyke in forme to matter, saue that it is moare duly knyt together then is matter, and doth not smell so euyll as it: or els you may lyken it to thynne fleame. This ground is then grosse when the veynes are replenyshed with raw humoures. Howbeit, this grossenes or thyckenes is not alwayes an euyl token. For sum=tyme it is a sygne, that nature hath pre uayled agaynst the crude humoures, which caused dyseases, and doth expell soch superfluous excrementes. & that shall you dyscerne, by the goodnesse of the colour, and also if it cum in the de= clynyng of the syckenesse: for if it cum at the begynnyng, other in the increase of the syckenesse, then are they to be suspected as euyll: especially if they bryng with them euyll coloures.

A thynne grounde, beyng also pure, & so cleuyng to the bottom of the vrinal, that it wyll not lyghtly ryse, though the vrynall be shaked, is a tokē of great weakenesse of nature in the thyrd con= coction, & soch a ground appereth most

in

Grosse grounde

Thynne grounde

OF VRINE. 40.

in whyte & watery vryn. Howbeit sum tyme a thynne grounde cumeth by the reason that the raw humours are extenuate, thorough naturall heate, which gettyng new strength, doth extenuate & disperse all grossenes of raw humors within the vaynes. For the propty of hete, is to knyt & bynd together thynn thynges, and to extenuate & dysperse grosse & raw thynges. Now as touchyng the coloures of the ground, the perfecte grounde ys nother excedyng whyte, nother yet pale, but meane betwene both: for if there appere any soch excessyue whyte, thē is it sum ragge of phlegmatyke mater, other els matter extremely cōcocted, which cumeth frō sum inward member beyng sore: & that may you dyscerne (as I sayd before) by the toughnes, & by the sauour. And if any man be desirous to know the cause why the groūde is whyte of colour, let him remēber, that y͏̄ groūd is the superfluous excrement of blood beyng perfectely cōcocted in the vaynes. Now that the blood it self, when it is exactly concocted, is turned into a whyte, or at least, a partye whyte coloure, you

Coloure of the ground

THE IVDICIALL

you may coniecture by the generation of mylke, and also of the sede of man, yea, & of matter, which all thre ar no thyng els but blood, exactly concocted saue ỹ matter compth of euyl blood. And therfore when so euer the ground hath in it any other colour thẽ whyte, it is no good tokẽ : as fyrst if it be pale

Pale.
Flaxen.

& flaxen coloured, then is it swarued from his right & commendable colour. How be it, yet it may be borne, as but meanely euyl, bycause that that colour cummeth of small excesse of choler.

Safren.

But if it be more hygher coloured by choler, so that it be saffren coloured, then is it an euyll token (as Actuari' sayth) for it declareth that choler is ex= cessyuely increased, other by the order of the dyete, other els by the corruption of the blood, other sum other wayes.

7. Aphor. 32

How be it Hippocrates in his Apho= rismes, semeth to say the contrary : for he sayth, that when the grounde is so coloured of choler, especially, if at the beginnyng of the syckenesse it were watery to syght, then doth it betoken a quycke syckenesse : that is too say, as

Philothe'

OF VRINE. 41.

Philotheus expoundeth it, a sickenesse that wyll shortely be ended : & so it may iustly be called a good sygne. Not with standing as in this poynte it is a good token, in that it sygnifieth tht the dis= ease is nygh the ende, so it may be cal= led (as Actuarius calleth it) an euyll sygne, bycause it doth betoken a chole= ryke syckenesse, and that choler doth vnnaturally abounde. And if this an= swere doo nott content you, though it content Antonius Musa) than may you say more better (as I thinke) thus: that if the grounde be at the begynnig of the syckenesse coloured with choler, and so encrease (as Actuarius semeth to meane) then is it an euyll token in dede : for hyt declareth both the abun= daunce, and also the increase of choler. But if the grounde , at the begynnyug of a cholerycke dysease, were watery that is whyte and thynne , and after= ward turne to safren colour, which is the exacte colour of choler : other els to a yellow colour (which is sũwhat lesse choleryke) then is it a token that the coleryke mater, which before laye lur

G.j. kyng

THE IVDICIAL,

kyng in the body, both now begyn to a voyde: and so the cause of sycknesse, thus by nature expellyd, health must nedes followe. As contrary wayes, if after yellow or saffren colour, it chaüge vnto whyter, and there be no certayne token of concoction, then is it an euyl sygne, and a token of phrensy. Howbeit, if there be any tokyn of certeyne concoction, then is the same a good sygne, so that if you take hede, you may parceyue here what a necessarye thyng it is to obserue order, in the alteratiõ of vrin / of which I haue partlyu spoken before.

Claret coloure. Red. Bloddy.

Now therfore to go forth yf the grounde be of claret coloure, other red or blew, the token is nott good. for these blooddye coloures cum other of to moch abundaũce of blood, other els by reason that the retentyue power is so feble, that it can not kepe in y͘e good humors, but suffreth them to run out.

Claret. Redd.

Claret colour & red, do betokyn a certain defaulte of cõcoction in y͘e vaines, & that thorough the excesse of red choler. But yet this defaute is but meane, and

OF VRINE. 42.

and without daunger, seyng that the hurte is onely by quantytie, where as sum other do hurte both by quantytie and qualytie also.

Bloddy.

Blooddye groundes are all together worse then red (though they be better then ashecolouryd, and blacke) for they betoken that the blood is nothyng duly wrought, especially if their quantytie be moche with all / for then the quantytie of mater doth let the powers to worke. whiche thynge yet as it may be borne, so it declareth nede of long tyme to recouer health.

But if this doo cum thorough weakenesse of the powers in them selfe, then is it an extreme euyll sygne: for it betokeneth that the powers are ouercum with werynesse in workyng, and be not able to kepe in the good and profytable humoures. whiche thynge to discern more exactly, you shal take artificial coiecturis, by other circūstaūcys, which geue also tokyns of iudgement: namely, as by the age of the persone, by his order of dyete, and soch lyke.

 Now to make an ende with the o-
    G.ij. ther

THE IVDICIAL

ther colours which ar of a darke hew: as blew, ashcolour and blacke. These of al other ar the worst, & most enmious to nature: and the nearer they cleue to the bottom of the vrinal, the worse thei are. These coloures cum of a blacke melancholy humour, beyng ingendred within the veynes, or els cūmyng frō sum other parte into them: other els it betokeneth deadly mortifyeng. But sumtyme it cummeth of sore bruſyng & stripes, & generally it cūmith (namely the blacke) other of excessyue colde other els excessyue heate.

And now for a conclusion what so euer I haue sayd of the grounde, you shall vnderstande the same to be spoken of the swymme, and the cloude / for they are in kynde but one thyng, saue that they dyffer in lyghtnes and hefte: and therfore also in places, but the iudgement of their substaunce, and colour is moch after one rate, though sum dyfference there be, as you shal here anon. And lyke wayes of their quantytie, which as it is then only commendable whē it is meane, so if it be greater then a meane

Blew.
Ashecolour
blacke

Quantytie.

Great.

OF VRINE 43

a meane, it doth declare sum alteration in man, though not alwayes extremely euyll. For sumtyme it is a token of fattyng, or growyng to a corporatenesse, and that doth it sygnify, if none other euyll sygne be coupplled with it. For though the persone fede moch on nourysshyng meates, and that with rest & an idle lyfe, yet naturall heate appereth so strong, that she can easely concocte soch meates. Accordyng to this sayth Galen in his Judicialles: that the plenty of the grounde in vryne betokeneth certayne & exacte concoction: and that as the body is replete w crude humoures, so it declareth y those same be in expellyng out at that preset tyme. And for this cause (sayth he) in all chyldren commenly, and in men also which fede moch, or be of sum other cause replete with humoures, their vryne hath a great grounde. Also often tymes it chauceth the pores of the skynne to be stopped / so that soche excrementes as were wonte to passe out by them, are inforced to seke a new passage, whiche they fynde most redyest by the vryne,

G.iij.   and

THE IVDICIAL

and thereof are the Contentes, and namely the ground often tymes encre=syd. And all these wayes chaunce in health. but in sycknesse, it chauncyth many & grosse superfluyties to appere in the vryne, as often as the naturall powers namely the alteratyue or con=coctyue power, beyng weakened, suche crude humours passe out vndefied. So doth it chauce (as wytnesseth Alexāder Trallian') that the vrin of them which haue the Collycke, is phlegmatyke, & hath a great groūd. But if the Cōtētes be other great, other grosse in ỹ begin=nyng, or in the augmētyng of sycknes, (namely if the paciēt haue any notable Ague) it arguyth abūdaūce of humors: to the concoction, of the whiche, there nedeth both strength of naturall pow=ers, with tyme & goode spede. And now contrary wayes must you iudge of the smallnesse of the Contentes : for they be caused other of great labour, longe fastyng, stoppyng or obstruction of the veynes, and such lyke partys, other els of slacknes of concoction and (as Ga=len sayth) when the body is replete w crude

Trall.li.3. cap.33.

Lytle Con=tentes.

Gal.2. pre=sag. Hip. 26

OF VRINE 44.

crude and raw humoures, then is the grounde great: but if the body be replenyſhed with choleryke humoures, then is there in the vrÿne other lytle groũd, oꝛ none at al: but in ſoch caſe it is well, if there be any ſublymation oꝛ ſwymme. Now ſemeth the place moſt meete to ſpeake of ſoch vꝛines as haue no ground at all, noꝛ other oꝛderly contente, and that wyll I do by the oꝛder of colours of the vꝛyne, accoꝛdyng as Actuarius pꝛocedyth.

Vryn with out ground

The vꝛyne that is very whyte, & exceding thinne, & ſo lacketh the ground, doth betokẽ other ſum notable obſtruction, otheꝛ immoderate cold, other els crudytie & lacke of concoction. And as theſe tokyns may be greater oꝛ leſſer, ſo ſhall the thynges whiche they betokyn, be iudged in lyke rate other moꝛe, other leſſer. But if the vꝛyn be pale coloured, oꝛ flaxen, and then lackyth Contentys, as it doth declare leſſer obſtruction, ſo it doth ſygnifye as great crudytie, as the other befoꝛe.

And ſo ſhall you iudge of vꝛyne that is Yellowe oꝛ Flaxen colowꝛed.

Giiij. Foꝛ

THE IVDICIALL

for in them it appereth, that naturall heate doth preuayle. Not with standyng soch thiges (I meane the defaute of the grounde with those coloures) may chaunce (as they often doth) thorough vehement payne, immoderate labour, long watchyng, & also defaulte of mater. But soch vrines as be higher coloured then these that I haue named, by their coloures they declare the qualyties of the humoures whiche doo preuayle, and also betoken a certayne putrefaction, & crudytie in the vaynes. It chaunceth also sumtymes, ỹ sum gethering sore being in sum of ỹ principal mēbrys, by his vnnaturall heate doth draw thether the mater (euē as it were by cuppyng) and so doth cause the vryne to haue no grounde. And though in dede it is neuer good token to lacke the grounde in a vryne, yet it is lesse to be complayned of, if the coloure & substaunce draw nygh to a meane: for in soch a case it betokeneth, that though nature be sumwhat slacke, yet wyll she shortely gether strengthe, so that there shall appere a grounde in the vryne.

Now

OF VRINE. 45

Now to shew you the reason, why it chaunceth no grounde to appere in the vrpne: fyrst in case of crudytie, when there wanteth parfect cocoction, there must nedes want also the contentes in the vrpne: for they ar the excrementes (as you myght say) and the superfluyties of the thyrde concoction. Lyke wayes though concoction be parfecte inough, yet may there want the contentes, if there be any notable obstruction or stoppig of the vaynes, namely seyng the cōtentes ar sumwhat grosse of substaunce, and therfore vnable to passe if the waye be any thyng stopped. After the same sort shal you iudge of long fastyng and defaute of meate, and more ouer of soch meates as ar vnapte to concocte. For in all soch cases there can be engendred few or no contentes. And contrary wayes though nature do worke many superfluyties, yet if ỹ wombe be so louse that it peldeth many seges, then as the vrin shal be the lesser, so shall the contentes be few or none: for nature then doth expell by sege those superfluyties, which
G.v. shuld

THE IVDICIAL

shuld cause the Contentes. And lyke wayes, when there is in any parte of the bodye an inflāmation, or excessyue heate, which doth draw mater to it, other that any of those partys ar weake vnto whiche nature is wonte to expell soch superfluyties: for in all soch cases there may want the grounde & thother contentys in the vryn. And as for sum of them (J meane crudytie & opilation) they may be well inough borne with all, vnlesse their contynuance be long.

But now agayne, there is great difference touchyng the tyme of the syckenesse in which it chauncyth: for in the begynnyng and increase of sharpe Agues, if the grounde be lackyng, it betokenyth great weakenesse of naturall strength, which vnneth may contynew vntyll the cheefe strength of the syckenesse. And after soche an vryne, there doth follow moche wakyng & dysquietnesse, halfe madnesse & troble of mynd. and all those shall be accordyng to the greatnes of the Ague, other extreme or mylde. And sumtime it is a tokyn that there shall be a getheryng sore in sum parte

OF VRINE. 46.

parte of the body, namely if other agreable causes cum therewyth, as a wynterly dyspofytion of the ayer, with an vncerten state of sickenesse and vnconstante alteration, and meane weakenesse of the pacyentys power. but in the declynation of the syckenesse, soch vryn ought not gretly to be blamed, for then hath nature escaped the bronte of syckenesse, though she be pet weake. Yea, and in the cheefe strengthe of syckenesse (as well as in the declynation) it may seme no straunge thyng, if nature (as though all redye she had the ouer hande) doo gether hyr power together, and drawe a lytle nouryshement to hyr selfe, and thereby causyth lytle or no ground to appere. But after warde when she is sumwhat refreshed, and doth more lyberally nouryshe the body, then doth she shew furth contentys in the vryne. And lyghtly the order of the cōtentes is soch, that fyrst there appereth a cloude, whiche afterward doth gether more strong and weyghty substaunce, & doth becum a swymme or sublymation: & last of all when it hath gethered

THE IVDICIALL

gathered a ryght naturall whytenesse, and dew substaunce, then wyl it grow to a grounde.

Of dysforme Contentes. The .9. Chapiter.

Other thiges shuld I here speke of as touchyng the Judicial of the contentes, both of their stabylnesse, that is, their contynuaunce in good forme, and of their dew knitting, beyng nother tattered and dysparsed, nother yet ouer moch clodded togeder: But bycause the exacte iudgemēt therof excedeth the capacite of meane wyttes (for whose sake I haue wrytten this boke) and can not lyghtly be percepued of them, but by thinstruction of a lyuely voyce, I wyll for this tyme ouer passe the exacte and perfecte declaration of them, reseruyng it to a place more dew / and now wyll I brefely ouer runne the other thynges which remayne to be consydered in vryne / but yet not without sum mention of those other, as occasyon cummeth: and fyrst those dyfforme Contentes which occupye the place of the ground, & therfore take

Dysforme Contentes.

OF VRINE 47

take his name also. Of this sort there
are .iiij. principall: the fyrst is in byg=
nesse of a small fatche, & red coloured,
which you mai cal therfore red fatches,
bycause of their lykenesse. These (as
wytnesseth Galen) ar engendred of the
consumption and wastyng of the flesh,
when the fattynesse is all redy molted
away. But in this there is great dyf=
ference, for sumtyme it is only the wa=
styng of the reynes, and sumtyme of
the hole body: as if there appere in the
vryne tokens of dew concoction, then
is that waste in the reynes only. But
if there appere in the vryne defaulte of
concoction (namely beyng great) or if
the pacient haue an Ague, then is it
the waste of the hole body, & that stan=
deth well with reason, that when it be=
tokeneth the waste of the hole body,
there must nedes appere defaulte of
concoction: for in soch case those par=
tes which ar the instrumentes of con=
coction are so weakened, that they can
not do their offyce. These Contentes,
by reason that they are grosse & heuy,
therefore they appere alwayes in the
bottom

Red Fat=
ches.
6. Epid.

TEE IVDICIAL

bottom of the vrinall. Other difforme cōtentes there be also, of which sum ar lyke branne, and sum lyke scales. And of those that are lyke branne, there is one sorte smaller, and in other grosser: the smaller sorte is lyke the branne of Wheate that is fynely grounde, and those maye I call fyne Branne. The grosser is lyke branne of barley, or of euyll grounde wheate, and may there= fore be called grosse branne, for it is thryse as bygge as the other.

 The thyrde sorte which is lyke sca= les hath no notable thyckenesse, but onely bredthe and lengthe. These thre do betokyn waste of ẙ strongest partys of the body: but yet not all a lyke, as Hippocrates doth declare in the secōde boke of his Prognostykes. How be it bycause that place of Hippocrates is so diffyculte, that scarsely the great ler= ned men can agree theron, I wyll not now medle therewith, but wyll wryte Actuarius mynde of those thre.

When the Ague (sayth he) is groun= dyd in the bottome of the veynys, then there apperith soch fyne branne.

        How

Brannye contentys.

Fyne bran.
Grosse brā

Scales.

Fyne bran.

OF VRINE. 48.

How be it sumtymys it is a tokyn of thonely greefe of the bladder beynge scabbed, as wytnessyth Hippocrates iiii. Aphor .lxxvij. But then hath the pacyente no Ague, and agayne there doth appere tokyns of concoction in the vryne. But when it cummyth of the hole body, this is the cause therof. The Ague gettyng onys and preuay= lyng vnto the harde partys of the body (as in those Agues whiche are called Feuers hectyke) then in the strypyng betweene those partys, and the Ague, the Ague hauyng the mastery, doth by his violence rase of soch brānye scurfe. For the nature of fyer (whose operatiō the Ague hath) is to worke accordyng as the mater is, that hyt findeth, other to molte it, if it be a lyquyde and vn= ctuouse thynge, other elles to scale it and frette it, if it be harde and vnply= aunte: and the harder that the mater is, the greater scales it frettyth of: which thing you may se by dayly expe= rience: how fier molteth waxe, & tallow and soch lyke, turnynge them into ly= quydes: wheras of pryn and other me= tals, it makyth scales and not lyquore.

THE IVDICIALL

Scalys.

But whan the Ague hath atteyned, & ouer sette, not only the substaūce of the vaynes, but also the stronge partes of the body, and doth molt & waste them, then doth ther appere in the vrin, scales, brode and thynne, which you shall know to cum of the hole body (as I said of the other before) if the paciente haue an Ague, other there appere defaulte of concoction in the vryne / elles if these .ij. be absent, it may cum of the blysteryng of the bladder, as Hippocrates wryteth .iiij. Aphor .lxxri. and namely, if there be in the vryn an euyll sauour with all. Now to speake of the great and grosse Branne, which as it is moche greater then the other, so it doth declare a greater strength of the Ague, and that in the hole body, and al the partes of it, enflamyng & burnyng the hole substaunce thereof, & therfore is it nott onely the worst of them all, but is nygh vnto a deadly sygne: and that other by the waste & consumyng of the great & strongest partes of the body, or els by the burnyng or dryeng vp of the blodde. Which .ij. thynges you

Grosse branne.

OF VRINE. 49

you may discerne a sunder by the co=
lour of them. For if they be redde, then
cum they of the burning of the bloodd:
but if they be whyte, then cum they of
the waste of the strongest partys of the
body. Of this kynde of Contente spe=
kyth Hippocrates, sayeng : In what
so euer Aguys there doth appere grou̅=
dys, lyke vnto grosse Branne, it is a
tokyn that the syckenes shall contynew
long. Which sayeng Galene doth vn=
dersta̅d so to be true, if the pacient haue
suffycient strengthe to contynew with
soch syckenesse, els it may be a signe ra=
ther of shorte lyfe, then of long sicknes.
For as the tokyn is commynly dedly,
so those few that do escape, do recouer
hardly, & not without long sufferaunce
of the vyolence of that cruell Ague.
Now as touchyng the foreknowledge
of it, whether the pacyent may endure
with it or no, that shall you gether of
the multytude order, and stablenes, or
vnstablenesse of it. For if they be ma=
ny in nomber, & procede to worse and
worse, then is it an euyll and mortall
sygne, and doth declare that nature is

Hippoc .7.
Aphor .31.

H.j.   weryed

THE IVDICIAL,

weryd, & doth quyte faynte, thorough the waste & decay of the hole cōstitutiō of the body. But contrary ways if thei appere few, & do alter cōtynually vnto lesse euyll tokyns, then is there good hope of health. and this shal suffyce as touchyng these. Now to speake of the rest, as of raggyd scrappys, herys, and other lyke. Fyrst you shall vnderstand that sumtyme a good grounde is cou=pelyd with certen euyll & vnconcoctyd fragmētes of al sortes of humours. for sumtyme there apperyth with the con=tentys certein raggyd scrappys, encly=nyng in colour toward a yellow, other a whyte, or els sum soch lyke. yf those appere in great quantytie, they declare the mater to be halfe vnconcocte, and that that humour (whose scrappis thei are) doth abound in the depthe of the body, & is adust or burnyd. but if they be few, thē declare they $\stackrel{e}{p}$ malice of the humour to be mylder, & that $\stackrel{e}{p}$ vse of e=uyl meates doth cause them. the greter that soch raggyd scrappes ar, the lesser adustion of humors they declare to be in the vaynes . & the lesser they be, the greater heate they do betokyn. for the

Ragged scrappes.

OF VRINE. 50.

cause of soch raggyd scrappis, is excessyue heate, which doth turne those humours into a thycknes, & as it were a bony nature, bi reasõ that they haue remainyd lõg in certen veines, & wer nother dissolupd, nother extenuatid, nother yet quyckly expellyd by vryne. Besydes these there ar herys of sundry lẽgthes, sũ an ynche, & sum an handful lõge, sũ loger, & sũ shorter: & these ar in colour whytely, & do betokẽ grefe of y͞e raynes. These ar ingẽdrid in y͞e water pipes, which go frõ y͞e reines to y͞e bledder, so that as lõg as those water pipis ar ĩ length, so lõg may those heris also be: which are a grosse & bakyd humor, wrought ĩ forme of a here. Of these spekyth Hippocrates, sayẽg: In whose vryn so euer ther doth appere lytle pesis of fleshe, other as it were heris, those same cum frõ the reynes: namely if the vryn be thycke. Howbeit these ar sũtimis sene ĩ soch mens vrines as fele no grefe in the reines, but onle haue fed sũ cõtinuĩg space on phlegmatike meatys which wil ppare mater to soch diseases as thei do also to many other grefes, of

Herys.

4. Apho. 76

H.ij. which

THE IVDICIAL,

which to speke in this place it is mete. But to go on with this thyng that we haue in hãd, besyde soch ragged scrappes and herys (as I haue spoken of) there appere sumtymps in the grounde of the vzyne, & also dysperkelyd abzode in the vzyne it selfe, sundzy and duyers kyndys of motys (as it were) whiche do declare that there is greefe dyspersyd in sundzy partys of the body. And this now may suffyce, as touchĩg contētis of eueri kinde: therfoze now wyl I a lytle repete out of Actuari' of the dyuersytie of iudgement by the placys oz regyons of the Contentys.

Motys.

The placys of the Contentys

The lowest regyon

That grounde which fleetyth nygh to the bottom of the vzynall, beyng in other poyntys also good and mylde, doth betokyn no straunge thyng. But if it be vnconcocte and diffozmyd, it betokenyth defaute in nature. And if his partys be dysparkelyd a sunder, it betokenyth a dulnesse in nature, whiche doth not respst the rebellion of noysum humozs. so that in soch case there apperyth nede, both of long tyme, and also moze strengthe to ouercum that euyll.

But

OF VRINE 51

But as it is commendable that the grounde fleete nygh the bottom of the vrynall, so is it dyscommendable yf it lye flatte on the bottom of the same.

Now as touchyng the swymme or sublymation, if it be good in coloure & other wayes, then doth it dyffer onely in place from a right ground / and that cummith of an vnnaturall wyndynes, which makyth it to be so lyght, and to fleete aboue his dew place: but if his co lour & lyke other poyntes be euyll, yet then doth it betokyn lesse euyll then yf it were in the right place of the groud. But now as touchig the thyrd & high= est regyon, whiche is the place of the cloudys: yf there appere a lyght and thynne cloude, it betokenyth no small greefe of the hedd. But this difference is there in the cloudys: the better that they be in coloure and substaunce, the farther they dyffer from a ryght good and naturall Content. & therfore nede they longe tyme to returne ther vnto. And contrary wayes: the worse that they are in colour and substaunce, the lesse they are to be blamyd by reason of

The middle regyon

The highest regyon

H.iij.   their

THE IVDICIAL

their place, which is so moch dystaunt from the naturall place of Contentys. for this is a generall rule : The lower that good contentys fleete in the vryn (exceptyng alwayes soche as cleue to the harde bottom) the better they are. And contrary ways of eupl contentis, & soch lyke, the hygher they fleete, the lesse eupll they betokyn.   Now to make an ende of this, you shal obserue a certayne proporcion that is betwene the partys of the vryne, & the partys of mannys body. the hyghest parte of the vryne doth betokyn the hyghest parte of the body, namely the hed, & soch other nere vnto hit. the myddle regyon of the vryne, doth represent the myddle partys of man : as the brest, the bowels and the partys about them. the nether regyon of the vryne doth purporte the lowest partys of man, from the bowels downe ward. And if you marke well this proporcion, you may the easyer iudge the grefes of the partys of man. For when the contentys which in co= lour & substaunce are naturall, & yet by the abundaunce of wyndynesse be lyfte
vp to

The proportion of the regions of vryne, to the partys of man.

OF VRINE 52

vp to the hygher parte of the vrpne, it declaryth sum great payne to be in the hed. And in lyke maner, when the swymme or sublymation doth declare grefe, that grefe must be iudged to be in the myddlemost partys of man : as I sayd before, and so of the other. Agayne, as this proporcion betwene the regions of vrpne and the partys of mannys body, doth declare the place in certayn heyght, so doth it in bredthe also by lyke proporcion, if you do duly marke ye syde vnto which ye contētys do declyne. And if you marke well what I haue sayd, you may perceyue that ye only cause of most soch grefis, whē the contentys is only dysorderid in place, cūmeth of an vnnatural windynes : but yet comenly annexed to phlegmatike & vnconcoctyd mater. And as this wyn= *Bubbyls.* dynes doth cause dysorder in the con= tentys, so it causeth also an other kinde of thinges not to be neglectyd in vrpn, & that is bubbils : which sūtymes flote in the ryng or garlād only, & sūtymes in ye middes of the vrpn only, & other ty mes do couer the hole face of the vrpn.

H.iiij. The

THE IVDICIAL

The bubbyls which stand rounde a bout ouer the garland only, and contynew without partyng, if they be of the same colour that the vryne is, they declare great payne to be in the hed : and that in al partys of the hed, if the bubbyls ioyne together without partyng. But and yf they occupy onely the one halfe of the garland, then is the payne in the one halfe of the hedd / & so furth may you iudge by lyke proporcyon.
But if they do parte in sundry placys, and ioyne not al together, it is a tokyn that the paine is the lesser, & cummyth of a weaker cause. The more yellower that their colour is, the greater they declare the payn in the hed to be. If they be whyte, or rather whytysh, & stande about in the compasse of the garland, they betokyn lytle payne or none. And yf the vryne be thynne with all, they betokyn weakenesse of naturall heate : or els the oppilation and stoppyng of the raynes, namely if there appere no ground in the vryne. This doth Hippocrates wytnesse, sayeng : When in the vryne there swymmyth bubbyls, they

7. Apho. 34

OF VRINE. 53.

they betokyn greefe in the raynes, and also that it shall longe contynew. The reason of the longe contynuaunce (as Galene & Philothe' do both declare) is bycause that the greefe cummyth of colde and tough phlegmatyke mater, which alwayes is longe before it may be ouercum. Plinye also sayth, that that vryn is euyll, which is full of bub= *Lib.28. ca.6* byls & thycke : in which, if the ground be whyte, it is a tokyn that there shall be greefe other about the ioyntes, or els about the bowels. Howbeit, yet sumtymys the bubbyls ar not an euyll tokyn, but contrary wayes a good to= kin of concoction, and declare that na= ture doth now apply hyr self wholly vn to concoction. and this do the bubbyls sygnify, when they appere in that wa= ter, in which they were not sene longe before. and therefore in an Ague, we may coniecture the declynation of it, when we se bubbyls to appere after that sorte : excepte it be so, that they apperyd in the vryne at the beginnyng of the syckenesse, & hath so contynuyd styll : For then they declare greuouse

H.v. payne

THE IVDICIAL

paine to be in yͤ hed, yea & that daūge=rous if yͤ vrin also be thin in substance. but if the substaūce of yͤ vryn be thicke, then the bubbils ar not so euyl a signe, nother declare so greuous daunger.

Fome.

Sumtymes in the stede of bubbyls which do not appere when they shuld, it sufficith yͤ there appere a grosse fome, (as it is sūtimes sene to rise vpō wyne) & it doth betokē euen yͤ same thing that the bubbyls do, especially in yͤ declina=tion of yͤ ague, of which I spake a lytle rather. These bubbyls do appere very thycke about the garllād, in the vryn of him that hath yͤ ysshew of rede, or waste of nature. Sūtymes also there ar sene in yͤ bubbyls certein small scrappes (as you wold say) moch lyke heris in grosse nes, & of soch lengthe sūtyme that they reche frō the one syde of yͤ bubble vnto the other. & sūtymes lōger, & sūtymes shorter. which thinges may cum other of the wastyng of the reynes, other els of the sheding of nature. The cause of the generation of bubbyls, and also of the dyspersyng and eleuation of the contentes, is an vnnatural wyndines. of which, as there are dyuerse kyndes

OF VRINE. 54.

moch differig a sunder, partely in mul=
tytude, partely in substaunce, & partely
also in qualitie. so doth the bubbyls en=
gendrid of them, dyuersely vary, accor=
dyng vnto those dyfferencis, whether
thei be sole & seueral, other iointly men
ny knyt together. But wyndynes, if it
be grosse, then doth it puffe vp soch bub
bils / & if it be subtile, thẽ doth it rather
worke a dyspertion in the contentes, &
is not able nor meete to cause bubbyls.
and hereby may you know the qualitie
of the wyndynes, & lyke ways also the
quantitie. For ther appereth lesse quã=
tytie of wyndines to be, where the con=
tentys onely are dispersyd, then where
soch bubbyls be engendred. Now as
touchyng the other qualyties of it, as
heate & colde (which ar ẙ chefe qualites
in dede, & most actyue) you may iudge
them by the colour of the bubbyls. for
as pale colour & other low coloures de=
clare coldenes of that wĩdines, so high
coloures enclynyug towarde yellow or
hygher, be certen tokyns of heate.
Bubbyls that ar small, & thycke knytt
to gether in the garlande of the vryne,

doth

THE IVDICIAL

doth betokin a grosse windines, whose cause can not easely be vaynquyshyd / for the grossenes & toughnesse that is in them, wyll not suffer them to swell great, and that causyth them to be so small. And contrary wayes, the greter that the bubbyls be , and the moare boullid, the more they declare that wyn dinesse that causyth them to be feuerid from toughe mater. More ouer, the colder that soch wyndynesse is, yͤ lesser greefe is felte of them.

Bubbyls in the vryne of olde men, namely beyng great and large, doo be⸗ tokyn colde wyndynesse : but sumtyme soch bubbyls ar a sygne of a rewme de⸗ stillyng from the hed into the lyghtys, especially if the pacient at the entryng of somer were very hotte , and so dyd drinke moch , whiche mater, the hedd beyng dryed dyd draw vnto hym, and dyd destyl agayne parte of it downe in to the lyghtys, whereof cummyth a cough, and parte of it, into the wombe, which therby is moued to laxe.

Of the garland & other lyke thynges.

As

OF VRINE. 55.

AS I haue compendiouſely, and yet not very ſlyghtly ſpokyn of thoſe former partys, to be conſyderyd in vrin: ſo wyll I brefely ſpeke of a few more, whiche may not be well omyttyd, and ſo make an ende of the Judiciall. Fyrſt therfore in the ouer parte of the vrin, round about the edge of the vrpne there apperyth a garland, circule, or ryng, whiche doth there appere, by reaſon that the hygher parte of the vrpne beyng thinner then yͤ reſt, and more ſubtyler, & therfore doth not onely more ſoner alter, but doth alſo more redyler declare that alteration. howbeit ſumtyme there doth appere no ryng at all: and that is, when the coloure of the vrpn, & of it, is all one, by reaſon of yͤ great force of that cauſe whiche alteryth the vrpne: but yet ſo that nature doth matche that humour, and is nother ouercummyd by it, nother yet hath ouercum it. For if nature haue playnly other gotte the victorpe, other loſt it, then is there an other coloure in the garland, then is in the reſt of the vrpne. Nowe if the coloure of the

The garlãd

THE IVDICIAL

the vryne be euyll, & the coloure of the garlande better, it is a tokyn of health: as if the colour of the vryne be yellow, red, or crymsen, or any soch lyke, & the colour of y̆ garlãd be whyte, or whytely, it is a tokyn full of good hope: but when the coloure of the hole vryne is euyll, and the coloure of the garlande worser yet, then is hit an euyll sygne: As when the coloure of the vryne is greene, or purple, and the garlande worse colouryd, then is it a playne tokyn that nature is ouer cum, and that the euyll humoures haue gottyn the ouer hande.

Of these moze particulerly doth Egidius entreate but yet not moze truly nor moze suffyciently / his wordys are these: If y̆ circule of the vryn be thick and watery, it is a tokyn that the hynder parte of the hedd is oppressyd with phlegmatyke mater: but if it be purpyll colouryd and thycke, then is the foze parte of the hedde ouer chargyd with bloode. A pale and a thynne cyrcule declaryth the lefte syde of the hedd to be troublyd with melancolye mater:
but

OF VRINE. 56.

but if it be redde and thynne, it betokenyth choler to abounde in the ryght parte of the hedde. A leddy or asshe colouryd circule doth sygnifye the Fallyng Euyll, thorough the great greefe of the brayne, and farther declaryth that soche greefe shall procede by the senowes into the other partys of the bodye. but if after soch a leddye colour there followe a reddysshe coloure, that is a good tokyn: for then doth nature gether strengthe agayne, and the powers of the brayne reupupth.

If the coloure of the garlande be greene, and the pacyente haue a burnyng Ague, it is to be fearyd left that the aboundaunce of choler shall cause a Phrenesy.

Blacke coloure in the circule doth sumtyme betokyn mortifycation, and sumtyme onely extreme heate. but these shall you distincte (as I sayd before of the vrpne selfe) by the order of the colourys. for if greene coloure went before, then doth the blacke betokyn adustiō thorough heate. but if his colour last before was asshe coloure, then is

it a

THE IVDICIAL

it a tokyn of death, cūmyng thorough the dominion of colde. and thys as touchyng the coloures may suffyce for this tyme. Sumtymps also you shall perceyue a quyuerpng and trembelyng in the garland, & that declaryth greefe in the backe bone: and this menny to=kyns be takin of the circule or garlād.

Fattyneſſe.

And sumtymps there wyll ap=pere fleetyng on the vryne a certayne scumme or fattyneſſe, sumtyme lyke droppes of oyle: & sumtyme lyke a thyn spyders webbe: and these both doo be=tokyn the moltyng of the fatte within the body, as Hippocrates wytneſſyth in his Prognostykes: how be it in his Aphorismes he doth aſſygne hyt as a tokyn of the greefe of the raynes pe=culyerly, sayeng: In whose vryn there fleetyth fattyneſſe, and that moche at onys, they haue payne in the raynes, but shall not long endure. This A=phorisme doth Galen vnderstand so to be true, if that fattynes appere quick=ly and moch at onys: els yf it cum by lytle & lytle with longer contynuaūce, so doth it nott betokyn waste onely of
the

7. Apho. 36

OF VRINE. 37

the fatte about the raynes : but rather thorough out y̆ hole body, which figne yet, is not alwaye euyll, excepte it conꝛ tynew longe. for if it contynew but a lytle whyle, it declaryth no great euyll.

Now to go furth with other fygnes. If the vryn haue a ſtynkyng ſauour, it is euer an euyll ſygne / for it doth betoꝛ kyn ſum putrefaction, moꝛe oꝛ leſſe : as of the bladder onely, by ſum blyſter oꝛ ſoꝛe in it : & that moſt certaynly, when the ſtynche is very great, and there apꝛ peryth alſo ſcales in the vꝛin, & matter. but if there be matter in the vꝛyne, and the ſtynkyng ſauoure but meane, then doth it declare the ſoꝛe to be in ſũ other parte of the body but this euer is true, that matter in vꝛyne is a tokyn of a ſoꝛe. and if in contynuaunce of tyme the matter and ſtynche doo abate, it is a good tokyn : but if they other contyꝛ new oꝛ increaſe, it is an euyll ſygne.

If the vꝛyne doo ſtynke, and there apꝛ pere no matter in it, then is it a tokyn of ſum moꝛtifyeng. For if there be in the vꝛyn meane tokyns of concoction, then is the moꝛtifycation in ſum one

Stinkyng ſauour.

J.j.   parte

THE IVDICIAL,

of the body: but if the other sygnes in the vryne be euyll, then is that morti=fication, rather of the hole bodye, then of any one parte of it.

And thus haue I ouer rūne brefely the cheife thynges to be consyderyd in vryne, which (I say) ar appertainyng or annexyd to the vryne it self. how be it two other thynges there ar, whiche though they be more playner thē these other, yet may they be ouer passyd no more then the other: that is to saye, blood cummyng furth with the vryne, and grauell expellyd therwith also.

Blood.   Blood cummyng furth with vryne, doth declare sum sore to be in y̆ raynes or bladder (as Hippocrates writyth in his Aphorismes) other els sum vayne to be brokyn about the raynes / name=ly if it cum sodenly, & without manifest cause. Howbeit, as Galen, Oribasi', and other dyuerse do declare, & reason also with experience, doth consent) there may appere blood in y̆ vryn also, if that there be soch a sore in the lyuer, or in the shafte. but in any of these ca=ses, the payne felte in the place, & parte

wyll

OF VRINE.   58

wyll vtter frõ whence ẏ blood cũmyth.

Now to speake of grauell, Hippo=
crates saith : In whose vryn there ap=
perith grauell in the bottom, they haue
the stone in the bladder, or elles in the
raynes, as Galen addith : but cõmenly
if the stone be in the raynes, the grauel
wyll be red, as Hippocrates declaryth
in his syrte booke of his Epidimies.
And thus now wyl I make an ende of
the Iudiciall of vryne.

Grauell.

*Of the commodyties & medicyns
of vryne. The .II. Chapiter.*

The greatest commodytie of vryne
is all redy declaryd: that is, that
hyt doth declare vnto man, the
menny folde diseases whiche happen
vnto him / and thereby, doth not onely
geue hym knowledge of the cause, and
so consequẽtly of the cure of the same/
but also warnyth him before of ẏ grefe
to cum, whereby he may take an occa=
syon to eschew it, if he wyll be diligent.
Now as this is the greatest cõmodite
of vryn, so it hath menny other as wel

I.ij.   in vse

THE IVDICIAL

in vſe of medicine as other wayes, of which I wyll wryte ſum, though not all. And firſt out of Plinie, which reſytyth ſtraunge operations of the vryn of a Hedgehogge, and of a beaſt, that yͤ Grekes cal Leontophonon, & more ouer of the beaſt Lynx, which I omytt now, with menny other: but this wyll I not ompt, that Hoſthanes ſayth: That if a man let his owne vryn drop vpon his feete in the mornynge, it is good agaynſt all euyll. And that it is good for the gowte, we may perceyue by Fullers, which neuer haue yͤ gowt: by reaſon that their feete are ſo often waſſhyd with it. The ſame Plinie wri tyth that the vryn of an Oſtryge, wyl do away blottys and moles of ynke. Alſo that if vryn be temperyd with wa= ter of lyke quantytie, and ſo powryd at the rootys of treys, it wyll both nou= ryſſhe them (as menny men ſay) & alſo dryue all noyaunce from them.

The vryne alſo of menne or of oxen temperyd with honye, & geuen to beis, wyll cure them that are poyſonyd with the flouer of the Cormier or Cornoiller tree.

Plinye.

OF VRINE. 59

tree. And lykewais if beanes be steppd in vrpne & water .iij. dayes before they be sowpd, some iudge that they wyl encrease excedyngly. Dioscorides sayth, *Dioscori=*
That a manys owne vrpne is good to *des.*
be dronke for styngyng of Adders, and agaynst poyson, and also agaynst the dropsp, when it doth begynne. and for the styngynge of see Adders, of Scorpions, and Dragons: it is good to soke the styngyd parte with all. The vrpne of Dogges is good to soke the place that is byttyn w a Dogge : & to clense maungynesse, and ytchynges, if salte peter be addyd thereto. and that that is olde wyl more strõgly clense scales, scurfe, scabbys, & hotte pusshys. Also it stayth frettyng sores, namely on the priuey members. Farthermore it stynchyth mattering eares, if it be droppid thereinto. and if it be sodde in the rynde of a Pome Granate, it expellyth wormys out of the earys. The vrpne of a Chylde vnder .xiiij. yeare of age, doth cure the toughnesse of breath , yf it be dronkyn. If it be sod in a brasyn vessell with honye, it healpth crepthys, & also

J.iij. the

THE IVDICIAL

the webbe & the tey in the eye / there is made of hyt & copper, good foulder for golde. The dregges of vryne is good for faynt Antonyes euyll, if it be noyntyd thereon: so that (as Galene doth wyfely adde) the fore be coolyd fyrst w sum other thyng, and be not burnyng. If it be hette with oyle of pryuet, and layde to the wombe of a woman, hyt wyll aswage the greefe of the mother, and curyth also the rifyng of the same. It clenfyth the eye lyddes, & the creythys in the eyes. Ore ftale beyng temperid with myrrhe, & droppid into fore eares, healeth the payne of them. The vrin of a wylde bore, is of y̆ same vertue, if it be kepte (as Sextus Platonicus writyth) in a glasse, & droppid warme into them: but it hath a more peculyer propertye in breakyng of the ftone, and to expell the same, if hit be dronke. Gotes vryne dronke euery day, with Spyckednarde, & .iij. ouncys of water, is good for the dropfy / for it expellyth vryne by the fege, & it curyth paine of the eares, if it be dropped into them. Affe pyffe (as it is writtyn) is
good

OF VRINE 60

good for the greefe of the raynes, if it be dronke.

Mulys stale (as Paulus Aegineta sayth) is good to heale payne in the ioyntes. The stale of Camels & gotes also, doth prouoke sege, & therefore is good for them that haue the dropsye.

Sextus Platonicus sayth, that Gotys vryne (if it be dronke (doth prouoke womans termys, and curyth payne in the eares beyng droppid into them: and beynge myrid with mulset wyne, and so droppid in the eares, it drawith out matter if there be any. *Sextus Plato.* *Paulus Aegineta.*

The vryne of a wylde Bore with mulset vyneger, is good for the Fal= lyng euyll, if hit be dronke.

A Dogges pysse temperyd with dust, and layde in wolle, wyll heale cor= nys merueloufely, & destroy wartys.

A Chyldys vryne wyll heale the styngyng of a Bee, Waspe & Hornet, if the place be washyd therewith.

A mannys vryne wyll clense the freckyls & spottys in the face. And if a womã can not be delyuerid of the af= ter burden, let her drinke mãnes vryn,

J.iij.   and

THE IVDICIALL

and she shall be delyueryd strayght.

Columella, Columella sayth, that the best dun=
gyng for yong shottys of treys is man=
nys vrpne, namely which hath stande
halfe a yere. For if you water vynys
or apple treys with it, there is no dunge
that wyll cause so moche fruyte as hyt
wyll do: and not onely that, but it cau=
syth also the sauour and the tayst both
Constanti= of y̌ apples, & of the wyne to be moch
nus Africa the better. Constantinus Africanus
nus, saythe: that the vrpne of a sheepe or of
an oxe, with sum hotte oyle, is good for
the greefe of the earys that cummyth
Vitalis of colde. Urpne (as Vitalis de Furno
sayth) frettyth, dryeth, and burnyth:
and is good for the greefe of y̌ splene,
if it be dronke, as Gentilis writyth.

The vrpne of a male Asse (as the same
Vitalis sayth) temperyd with nardus
doth encrease and preserue heare, and
as sum say (by the writyng of Mar=
M. Virgi= cellus Virgilius) vrpne is of no smal
lius. nouryshment: for dyuerse folke in the
tyme of dearth, haue ben preserupd by
thonely vse and drinkyng of hit. Also
Marcellus Marcell' the practicioner in the .xxvij
Chapiter

OF VRINE. 61

Chapiter doth wytnesse: that the vrin of a man is good for dyuerse dyseasys of the wombe and bowels, and namely for the collyke: bycause that partely iṅ prouokyng of vompte, and partely by occasyonynge of segys, hyt expellyth strongly all noysum humours. and for the same cause doth commen practicioners keepe hit yet styll in dayly vse. Wlderycke Hutten also wytnessyth, that he did dryue away the Ague aboue viij. tymes, with thonely drinkynge of his owne vryne, at the begynnynge of his syckenesse. And menny styll do vse the same practyse, and it prouyth well. Lyke wayes Marsilius Ficinus writyth, that menny men do vse to drinke vryne for the Pestilence: which thyng dyd Galen wryte long before him and also Paulus Aegineta. and do testifye also that it preseruyd them that dranke it: at the least way as they thought.

Vldericus Huttenus.

Marsilius Ficinus.

All vryne (as Galene wrytyth) is hotte in vertue, and sharpe (as sayth Aegineta) howbeit, it dyfferyth accordyng to theim that make it: For the hotter they ar that make it, the hotter

Galen.

J.v. is it

THE IVDICIAL

is it also, & lyke wayes the colder vrine cummeth of a colder bodye. Mennys vrin is the weakeſt of all other, excepte tame barrow hogges / for they in very menny poyntes agree with man : but the vrpne of wylde bores is ſtronger.

Mennes vrpn is of as ſtrong clenſyng vertue, as any thyng els / & therefore do fullers vſe it to ſcower & clenſe their cloth. And in cure of greefes alſo for the ſame reaſon, it is vſed to ſoke & waſſhe maunginesse, & ſcabbydnesse, and runnyng ſores that ar full of corruption and fylth / and specially if they haue in them putrified matter : and for ſoch ſores on the preuy members it is good, and for matteryng eares, & for ſcalles and ſcurfe, if the hed be waſhed in it. I haue healed with it menny tymes ſores on the toes, namely whiche came of bruſes, & were without inflãmation, & that in seruaũtes & husbãdmen, which had a ieurney to go, & no Phyſition with them / byddyng them to wette a ſmall cloute with it, and to put it into the ſores, & then to bynde a cloth about it / & as often as they lyſtid
to make

OF VRINE. 62

to make water, to let hyt fall on theire fore toes / & not to take the cloth away tyll hyt were quyte hole.

That medicyne whiche is made of Chyldes vryne, called of sum men, in Greke Chrysocolla (that is to sai, gold foulder) bycause men vse hit to foulder golde. This (I say) is excedyng good for fores that ar hard to heale: for this medicyne do I vse for the chefest, mixyng hit with soch other thynges, as ar good for soch lyke fores.

In the tyme of Pestilence, in Syria menny dyd drinke Chyldrens vryne and mennes also, and thought that they were preferued by hyt.

Of vryne also, doe Alchumystes make dyuerse thynges, as salte, and other thynges mo.

And mennye other commodyties there be of vryne: as for wasshynge and scouryng, and other lyke, whiche for breefenes I ouer passe / and the rather bycause they ar commenly knowen of all folke.

Of the dyseases touchyng vryne, and the remedyes for the same.

Now

THE IVDICIALL

Now to come to that I promysed as touchyng the greefes which hynder vryne, or expell it dysorderly, other in tyme oftenner then is meete, other in qualytie, with other facyō then is agreable to it, or lyke other sorte: I wyl breefely wryte, not entendynge too teache the arte of curynge them, whiche wolde requyre a longer treatyse, and a meter place. But onely to name certayne of the most commyn diseasys, and to sett after them soche symple & vncompound medicyns only, which cure those greefes. And though I wryte not now so largely as I onys entendid, another tyme I wyll recompence it. Fyrst therfore touchynge the *Stoppyng* hynderaunce or stoppyng of vryne: it *of vrine.* is not vnknowen that one cōmen cause *The stone.* is the stone, whiche sumtyme is in the raynes, and sumtyme in the bladder. I shewed you before, that commenly you mai disserne those two a sunder by the colour of the grauell: but the more sure tokē is ẙ greefe in the sycke parte.

Now for the cure of the same, doth these medicyns serue, whiche followe.

But

OF VRINE 63.

But as I haue alwayes sayd, you shall vse them w̄ the counsell of sum learned Physicion: for there is great difference both of the greefe, & of the medicyns.

Medicyns for the stone, both in the raynes and bladder,

Astra Bacca.
Ameos.
Sower Almondes.
Angle toches sodd
Betony.
Bryony roote.
Bylgrumme.
Chamamell.
Capers barke, namely of the roote.
Carret sede.
Clotte sede.
Docke roote.
Fenel: sede, & roote.
Gotys blood.
Gladyan.
Gromell.
Gumme of Plum tree, & Chery tree.
A hedge Sparow.

Harebell.
Kneholme roote and beryes.
Madder roote.
Hygh Malowes sede & roote.
Mogworte.
Perseley.
Pellyter of spayn
Pyony beryes. which ar black
Radyche.
Sampere.
S. Johns worte
Sperage.
Scholme.
Swynes Fenell.
Sothernewood sede.
Tente worte.
Tutsan

THE IVDICIAL

Tutsan beryes, Water plantayne, Wynter Gyllofer,

And besyde these, and dyuerse other, Also the stone it selfe that came from a man, beynge brayde & dronken, wyll breake & expell that other within him. Besyde the stone also hit chaunceth the vryne to be clene stopped, by reason of weakenesse of the expulsyue vertue, & sumtymes thorough cloddes of blood, which rest in the shafte, sumtymes also thorough tough & clammy humoures: and sumtyme thorough sum swellynge within the yarde, and dyuerse other wayes also, of whiche the declaration is to longe for this place & tyme: but an other tyme of them I entende too wryte at large, and of all other grefes of mānes body. But to returne to this mater that is in hand. One other stop of vryne there is, which doth not clene let hit, but causeth hit to auoyde lesser then it shulde: & this cummeth of lyke causes as that other laste dyd, saue that the cause is lesse, accordynge as y̆ stay of vryne is: & therfore the cure in both is moch lyke. For if it cum of we=
kenesse

OF VRINE. 64

keneſſe of the expulſyue vertue, then ẘ the vſe of other hotte meates & dẛikes, thoſe medicyns ar good, which do pɽo uoke vɽyne, as theſe be that follow.

Medicyns which do prouoke vryne.

Aniſe ſede. Laſe ſauery.
Alyſaunders. Lekes. Myntes.
Alkakengi. Margerom.
Baſyle. Maydenhere.
Bylgrũ. Pauew. Pepte.
Cammocke. Pegella Romana.
Charlocke. Pettle. Pepper.
Cheruell. Pye kpall.
Carawayes. Quynces.
Calamus aro=
maticus. Rew. Roſemary.
Rocquete.
Cubebes. Saupne.
Dictany of Cãdi Sage. Sauery.
Dɽagance. Tyme.
Fumytoɽye.
Fatchys. Ualeryon.
Flower delyce. Wylde margerom
Garlyke. Wylde Perſelcy.
Ground pyne. Wylde Tyme.
Gynger Water Creſſes.
Helecãpane. Woodbynde.
Honye.
Junip & ẙ beries   with

THE IVDICIALL

with menny other, and namely those
for the most parte, which I named be=
fore to be good for the stone. but there
must be discretion in the vse of them.
Besides these, is there a disease named
y̌ Strāgury (whiche sū corruptely call
the Stranguryon) in whiche dysease,
Excesse of vrine. the vryne doth contynually drop furth
as fast as it cōmpth into the bladder.
and therfore may it well be notyd the
fyrst kynde of soch greefes, as prouoke
forth, and forther vryne excessyuely.
For that Strangury, these medicyns
followyng are notyd good.

Medicyns for the Srangurye.

Alysaunder.	Sperage.
Astra bacca.	Seholme.
Brokelyme.	Spatula Fetida.
Ceder beryes.	Turpentine was=
Ceterake.	shyd.
Calam' aroma=	
ticus.	Wylde Fenell.
Gladyane.	
Knotte grasse.	Water myntis.
Kneholme.	

But you must consider (as I haue ofte
sayd)

sayd) that as the dysease may cum of sundry causes, so it must haue sundrye curys. For most cõmenly these ar good that I haue wrytten: yet such may be the cause of the sickenes, that they mai do harme / therfore take always counsell of sum learned Physition.

Another kynde of excessyue makyng of vryne cũmyth of the weakenesse of the retẽtiue vertue in yͤ raines / wherbi the pacient pysseth as fast as he drinketh, and that in lyke quantytie. This may I call the fluxe of vryn, or pissyng euyl: or after the imitation of the Grekes, the pysse gowte. For whiche dysease it is not greatly cõmendable to set furth medicyns wͭ thonly bare names. Howbeit, if I do hyt, I trust no man wyll the rather mysuse them / namely beyng warned so often to take no medicyns without counsell: & specially in this thyng: for sum of the medicyns must be receyued inwardly, and sum of them emplasterid outwardly.

Fluxe of vryne
Pyssynge euyll
The pysse goute

Medicyns for the pissyng euyll.

Apples. Cycorie.
Comferye. Dates.

K.j. Endyue

THE IVDICIAL,

Endyue.	Paritarye.
Elecampane.	Penny worte.
Lettys.	Perys.
Lyntels.	Pome granate.
Myrtell beryes.	Purselane.
Pyght shade.	Vyne leaues.

Other defaultes there be of excesse of vryne, as of them whiche can not kepe their vryne, and namely of chyldren, which pysse their beddes. This dysease cūmpth often tymes of the dissolution of that muscle, which shuld kepe in the vryne / & therfore requyreth cure meete for it, & vnmeete for this place, & soche shortenesse. Wherfore for this tyme, here wyll I make an ende, trustĩg that all men wyll with as gentle herte receyue this my wryting, as I of gentylnes haue takẽ ẏ paynes to set it forth.

Additions.

Of the dyuersities of coloures, and of the makyng of them.

Bycause that it is not very easy for euery mã to distincte colours duly a sunder, I thought it good at ẏ ende of this boke, a lytle to touche the distinctiõ & making of them, namely of soch as ar mẽtionid before ĩ this boke.

Mylke

OF VRINE. 66

Mylke whyte, by the name hit selfe doth sufficiently declare what it is: for hit is the very colour of mylke, though the substaunce nede not to be so thycke in the vryne, as in the mylke / for the colour must be vnderstand seuerall frõ the substaunce, both in this & all other coloures: whiche thynge wolde be remembred, for it myght els (as it hath often done) deceyue the symple folke. *Mylke whyte*

Horne whyte in lyke maner hath his name of ẙ thĩg that it assimilith most: for it is lyke the whyte & clere parte of a horne of a lanterne, or soch lyke. *Horne whyte.*

Gray, is lyke the whyte parte of a mānes nayle, nexte vnto the ioynte / or lyke hore here, that is not very whyte: for Gray is so moch darker then horne whyte, as horne whyte is darker then mylke whyte. *Gray.*

Pale colour hath a certayn apperaũce of yellow in it, but it is exceding lytle. If you seethe a pese of the rynde of Pome Granate, and then put to hyt thrice as moch cleane water, hyt wyll be a pale coloure. *Pale.*

But if you put therto lytle or none of clene *Flaxen*

K.ij.

THE IVDICIAL,

clene water, it wyll be flaxen coloured y̌ is sumwhat more yellower then pale.

Palewe   After it followyth pallew, which is a kynde of light yellow, sũ thing lygh= ter in colour then Crowne golde.

Yelowe.   For the colour of pure golde (as in an angell or royal) is a right yellow color.

Light saffrẽ   A lyght saffren, colour is that colour that saffren doth make when it is ste= ped in water, and layde lyght on any whyte. For if it be layde on depe, then doth it make a full saffren coloure. For

Saffren   that is called a saffren coloure, whych safferne doth dye, and not that, that is in the safferne it self. For that is a very

Red   red, and is hygher then claret, whiche
Claret   is a meane colour betwene safferne and red: as if it were made of them both myxed together.

Crimsyn   Crymsen is a darke bloody colour, well knowen by his owne name / but is not in vryne so lyght as it sheweth in

Purple.   cloth. Purple, nedeth not to be moch descrybed, beyng so cõmenly knowen / howbeit if you wyll see the makyng of it, myxe a darke crymsen w̃ an orient blew, and it wyll be a purple. And by=
cause

OF VRINE 67

cause that menny men be disceyued in the latyn name of this colour, you shal obserue that it is not that, which in latyn is called Purpureus colo2 (as most men thynke) fo2 that is rather a crymsen / but hit is called mo2e peculyerly Purpura violacea, o2 Passeus colo2.

 Blew coloure is the coloure of the cleare skye, o2 of asure. How be it in v2yne, it is not so o2ient: but if you wyl myx pure whyte (as whyte led, o2 pure lyme) with due po2tion of right blacke (as cole dust, o2 other lyke) then ther wyll of these, amount that blew, which is ascribed to v2yne. *Blew*

 Greene is a compownde coloure of blew & yellow duly temperid together, & the right greene haue J in this boke called a starke grene. But if the yellow do excede in it, then is it a light grene: and contrary wayes: if the blew do excede, then is it a darke greene. Of this greene doth Dioscorides meane, when he doth say of diuers herbes, that their leaues be blacke: and sumtyme when he noteth whytelynes to be in herbes, he meaneth a lyght greene / though o- *Grene*

Starke grene
Light grene

   K.iij. ther

THE IVDICIAL

ther tymes he vnderstandeth thereby a certen hozines / of which thig in myne Herball, you shall reade moze exactely.

Oyly. Oylye colours dyffer frō grene only in their lyghtnesse of hewe, & thynnes of substaunce in the vzyne, where they appere. The lyght oylye is sumwhat

Lyght. lighter (or rather bzighter & moze glitterynge then lyght grene. So is the

Starke starke oylye brighter then the starke

Darke grene / & the darke oylye, then þ darke grene, which all cummyth thorough the thynnes of substaũce in the vzyne.

Ashe colour Asshe colour is darker then blew, & is made of the same sorte as blew is, saue that it requyzeth moze of the blacke by two folde. this is the coloure of ledd, I meane in the vtter parte of ledde, which is moche darker then the ynner parte / though in dede both are one colour, & dyffer only in bzyghtnesse, and darkenes, which ought rather to be called the hewe of coloures, then colour.

Blacke Now as for blacke, I nede not to speake any whyt: for as all men doo know hit, so these very letters do shew hit / which though of all other hit be

the

OF VRINE 68

the moſt deadlye, yet is hit ſurely of all the moſt myghty: for hit ouer cũmyth all coloures, & none can chaunge hyt: ſo that well yt may be called the colour of death. For as death ouercummyth all bodyes, ſo blacke doth dampne all colours: beſyde that it is the meſſẽger & token of death, whiche is the ende of all thĩges, & blacke the end of colours.

Thexpoſytion of certayne wordes.

Now for bicauſe I was enforced to vſe ſum (though but few) termes in this boke, which be not well knowen of y̆ moſt ſorte of men, though a great nõber know them well ynough by oftẽ talkĩg w̃ Phyſitiõs, I thought it good here to declare ſum certayne of them, for the ayde of the moſt ſiple ſort.

Ages.

Bicauſe that in the iudgement of vrynes, the differences of ages ought to be cõſyderyd, you ſhall vnderſtand that the cheife differences of them are .iiij. that is to ſaye: Chyldehod, Youthe, Manhod, & Olde age / for though ther

R.iiij.   be com=

THE IVDICIAL

be comely .vij. Ages rekened, yet these be the .iiij. principall, & thother .iij. be comprehended vnder these .iiij. Chyldehod endureth from thower of byrth, vntyl thende of .xiiij. yeres of age, & is of complexiō hotte & moist. At thende of .xiiij. yeres begynneth youth, and lastyth tyl the .xxv. yeare / and thys age of all other, is in complexiō the most temperatest. From .xxv. yeres, vntyll .xxxv. yeres, is the flourishyng of māhod: but yet that manhod lasteth (though not in full freshnesse) vntyll .l. yeres of age / & this age is of complexion hotte & drye.

From .l. yeres forwarde, is the tyme of age peculyerly called / in whiche tyme mānes nature is colde & drye, and not moyst: as menny do falsely thynke.

Actyue qualities, se ye tytle of qualities. Alteratiue vertue, se in ye tytle of vtues.

Brightnesse in vryn must be marked for a seuerall thīg from clearenesse. For the brightnes betokeneth the oriētnes, & the bewty of the colour, w a certayne glisterpng. And clearenesse is referred to the substaunce of vryn, & is euer annexed to thynnesse of it. Yet is it a dy=
uerse

Childehod

Youth

Manhod

Age

Actiue. q.
Alteratiue
Brightnes.

Clearenes,

OF VRINE. 69

uerſe qualitie from thynnes. So may an vrpne be cleare in ſubſtaunce, by the reaſon of his thynnes/ & yet not bright in colour: & contrary wayes may an v= rpne be bright in colour, & not clere in ſubſtaunce / but this wold be well pon= derid, left this neceſſari diſtinctiõ cauſe an negligent confuſion.

Criticall dayes be ſoche dayes, on which there is (or may be) percepued ſum certayn token & great alteratiõ in the ſycke body, other to helth or death, or cõtinuaũce of ſyckenes. What theſe be, more at large I wyl hereafter (God willyng) declare in a booke peculyerly, bicauſe it requireth more largeneſſe of wordes, then is meete for this place. But one thing I muſt tel you, that the ſame daies alſo be called Iudiciall / but not Indiciall: for the Indiciall dayes are of an other kynde, but yet aſſociate to theſe other.

Crudite is the rawneſſe of the meate in the ſtomake, when p̃ natural opera= tiõ of it, can not duly diſgeſt the meate which it hath recepued: & therfore, the vrine which declareth defaulte of ſoche

K.v. digeſtiõ,

Crytical dayes.

Iudicial dayes

Crudite

THE IVDICIAL

digestiō, is called a crude, raw, & vncō=
cocte vryne. Cuppyng is so cōmenly
knowen, that it nedeth no declaration.

Cuppynge

Cloddy vryne

A cloddy vryne is that which hath
in it cloddes of blood, or other crude
mater, or any clusterynges of disformed
contentes. Darke groūde is not ment
of the darkenesse of colour, but rather
of the slendernesse of substāce, so that it
can scarcelye be dyscerned to be anye
grounde, by reason that hit is so neare
in shape & substaunce to the rest of the
vryne. Dulnesse of colour, is contrary
to brightnesse: so that when the colour
lacketh all brightnesse, then is it clene
dullyd. and what so euer thyng causeth
decay of soch brightnesse, that thyng
dullyth vryne. Those Contentys be
called diuerse, which haue nother their
owne ryght forme, nother any other
certen / but ar all together dysorderyd
and out of forme / rather sempnge to
be menny, then to be one.

Darke grounde.

Dulnes,

Dyuerse.

Duly knyt

Duly knytte, is a property of dew con=
tentes, when they are nott tatteryd,
raggyd, nor iaggyd, nor slytterynge a
sunder: nor yet ar not so clammyd to=
gether, as towgh fleme, or anye lyke

OF VRINE.

thyng : but are in a moderate meane betwene both these.

A getheryng sore, is that sore that is caused of the excessyue recourse of humoures into any parte of the body: as a byle, or any other lyke. *A getheryng*

Harueſt. seke Tymes of the yere. *Harueſt.*

Judiciall dayes: seke Critical dayes. *Iudiciall dayes.*

Inequalyte of substaūce ĩ vrin, doth appere to be ỹ diſformenes & diſagreīg of the partes of it together: as when it is thin in one parte, & thicke ĩ a nother. Howbeit, it is as well vsed for ỹ altera tion frō a meane substaūce to thicknes or thynnes, or other ways vnnatural. *Inequalyte*

Obstruction, is a stoppinge, com= menly of the vaynes and soche great cundytes (whiche conuaye bloodd or any other humoure) so that the thyng whiche they shulde conuaye, can not frely passe, as hyt ought. But if the lyke stopppnge happen in the pores of the skynne, (I meane those vn= sensyble holes, by whiche sweate paſ= syth out) so that nother swete, nor any lyke excrement may passe that wayes, then is hyt moast named Oppilation. *Obſtructiõ.*

Oppilatiõ

How

THE IVDICIAL

Howbeit, as these wordes be sumtymes vsed the one for the other, so they be applyed also to other sundry partes of the body: but euermore thei betoken soche stoppinge in that parte, that natures worke is hindered therby.

Principall membres

Principal members (as to our purpose now) are these .iij. the braine, the herte, and the lyuer.

Passiue
Putrefactiō

Passiue: seke Qualities.

Putrefaction is commenly knowen to signifie, rottynge.

Qualytyes

Qualyties actyue, ar named heate and colde, bicause they ar more apte & able to worke, thē to be wrought. And contrary wayes, drynes & moysture ar named passyue, or sufferyng qualyties, bicause they ar more redy to be alteryd by the workynge of heate and colde, then to worke themselfes: how be it, yet they do worke also.

The .4. tymes of sicknes

There be in sickenes .iiij. principall partes of tyme to be obserued of Physitians: The begynnyng of sycknes, the increase or augmentyng, the standyng or cheife force of it: & the declination or asswagyng of it.

The

OF VRINE.

The beginnynge, is from the tyme that sychenes hath ouer cum mannes strengthe, & brought him to lye down, tyll there do appere manifest sygnes of concoction of the mater, whereof the disease cummeth / at whiche tyme the sychenes waxeth fearcer & fearcer: and whyle it so cõtinuyth, that tyme is called the increase & augmenting of sickenesse: but when the violẽce of the sickenesse is at the most, so that the rage of it is at one stay, & nother incraseth nor decreaseth / that time is called the stãding stay, state, or cheife strengthe of ỹ sychenesse. And after that the furyous rage of sychenes doth abate and calme his cruell stormes, then is the declinacion of the sychenesse: after which (if the pacient escape, as very few dye in ỹ declinatiõ) then followeth recouerye to health againe. And these be the .iiij. generall or vniusall tymes of sicknes. Besides these ther be other tymes more pticuler, wherof now to speke I nede not. The diuersytie of tymes in ỹ yere ar duly to be obserued / for thei do moch alter mannes body.

The begin=nynge

The encrese

The state

Declinatiõ

Tymes of the yeare.

The

THE IVDICIAL

The springe   The Spring time encreaseth blood and bringeth al the partes of the body to a temperaunce, as nygh as hit can. For hit of all other tymes is the most temperate: nother excessiuely hotte, nor colde: nother moyst, nor drye. but of a iust temperature, as Galen proueth abũdantly ĩ his first boke of tempamẽt: where he doth moche blame them that name hyt to be hotte & moyst, whiche (he sayth) is of all other the most pe= stilent state of ayer. This spryng, after Galenes mynde, doth begynne aboute the x. day of Marche, & endeth aboute the .xxiiij. daye of Apryll: so that it la= styth but .vj. wekes & .ij. dayes. For at the rising of the Pleiades (whiche is

Sũmer   now in our tyme, about the .xxiiij. day of Apryll) he sayth that sũmer doth begynne. which sũmer is in complexiõ hotte and dry, & therefore meete to en=

Haruest   crease choler, which in that tyme doth abounde. The sommer lastyth .xxj. we= kes: Haruest doth begynne, after Ga= lenes mynde, aboute the .xvij. daye of September, and lastyth .vij. wekes.
The Haruest, is drye of complexion,
but

OF VRINE. 72

but nother oneli hotte, nor onely colde, but is distemperate in heate and colde. For in the mornyng & euenyng, hit is colde, & at noone it is hotte, so may it not be called iustly (as moast men doo name it) colde and drye. In this tyme doth melancholy encrease. At the ende of Haruest, about the .vij. day of No‑ uember doth Wynter begynne, which tyme is colde and moyst, and therfore encreaseth fleme, which is lyke in com plexion vnto hit. and the Wynter la‑ styth tyll the .x. day of Marche: so is it in length, about .xvij. wekes & a half: & then begineth the Spring tyme again. And this is the course of the yere, after Physicke. Other men which entreate of husbandrye, do parte the yeare into iiij. equall partes, geuīg .iij. monithys to euery tyme. Vnto the Spring, they geue February, Marche, and Apryll. to the Summer, May, June, & July. vnto Haruest, August, Septēber, Octo ber. & vnto Wīter, they appoynt, No‑ uēber, Decēber & January. Why the Physitiōs parte the yeare one ways, & wryters of husbādry anotherways, at more conuenient tyme I wyll declare.

Wynter

An other sort of these tymes.

THE IVDICIAL

Vertues
Attractyue

Alteratyue

Retentyue

Expulsyue

Vertues naturall ar .iiij, the fyrst is that which draweth nouryshment into dew places / & that is called the attractyue vertue. The second, is it that alteryth that nouryshment into a dewe forme to nourysh the body, & is called the alteratyue vertue. The thyrde, is that vertue, which kepeth in the good nouryshment, tyll the alteratyue vertue hath duly alterid it, & therfore is called the retentyue vertue : The fourthe, is called the vertue expulsiue, bicause his offyce is to expel those superfluous excrementes, which ar lefte when the other vertues haue done their offyce duly,

FINIS.

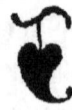

⁋ An vniuerſall Table for
Judiciall of Urynes.

The commoditie of Judgement by it.
The maner & ordre of Generatiō of v=
When the vrin ſhuld be taken. (rine.
What Urinall is beſt to this vſe.
What lyght, is beſt to ſee an vrine.
How longe it may be kepte before it be
That it ought not to be ſhaken (ſene.
   before it be iudged.
That it muſt bee kepte holy, and not a
   parte of it only,

⁋ Theſe thynges let iudgement.
   Moche ſhakyng of it.
   Darkeneſſe of lyght.
   Ouer bright lyght.
   The beames of the ſonne.
   Colde, and Wynde.
   A thycke or greene vrinall : & alſo
   if the vrinall be not due in faſſhiō

⁋ Theſe alter the vrine.
   Diuerſite of kynde. { Man. / Woman.

   Diſtinctiō of ages { Chyldhod. / Youthe. / Manhod. / Age.

THE TABLE.

Complexion. { Sanguine.
Cholerike.
Melãcholie
Flegmatike.

Diuersities of Contryes.

Tymes of the yere { Springe.
Sũmer.
Harueſt.
Wynter.

Meate and drinke.
Medicines, namely purgations.
Exercise and Rest.
Moche faſtyng.
Surfettyng and dronkennesse.
Moche watche.
Long ſlepe.
Anger.
Feare.
Company with women.
Great ſolublenesse.
Strong costyuenesse.
Moche vomyte.

⁋ These are to be conſydered
in Uryne.

i. The

THE TABLE.

i. The substaunce. { Thycke. / Meane. / Thynne.

ij. The quantitie. { Moche. / Meane. / Lytle.

iij. Clerenesse and darkenesse.

iiij. The sauoure.

v. The māner of pissig { With pain / With ease. / Willynge. / Unwillīg.

vj. Colours.
- Lightwhite. { Chrystallie. / Snowye. / Watery.
- Darkewhite. { milkewhite / Horny. / Grape.
- Pale.
- Flaxen.
- Pallew.
- Yellow or golde coloure.
- Safren. { Lyght safren. / Full safren.
- Clarret
- L.ij   Read

THE TABLE.

- Read.
- Crymsen.
- Purple.
- Blew.
- Greene.
  - Lyght greene.
  - grene as grasse
  - Starke greene,
  - Darke greene.
- Oylye.
  - Lyght oylye.
  - Starke oylye.
  - Darke oylye.
- Asshe coloure.
- Blacke.

vij. Cōtētes.
- The sedimēt, o₂ ground
- The sublatiō o₂ swime
- The cloude.

viij. The Crowne o₂ Circle.
ix. Bubbyls.
x. Fattynesse.

xj. Disforme cōtentes
- Hearys: lyke red ratchys.
- Brānny. grosse fyne.
- Scales.
- Ragged scraps
- Motes.
- Matter.

THE TABLE.

		Matter.
		Blood.
		grauel or stones
		Sede.

		Highest.
xij.	The Regions.	Myddle.
		Lowest.

xiij.   The ordre
xiiij. Continuaunce and alteration.

These in generall be the thynges meete to be considered in vrine, of whiche particulerly in this booke you may rede, as moch as to this tyme and purpose serueth, More largely haue J written thereof in a booke of the same tytle, but in the Latyn tonge, as more meete for learned eares, & for them that neede more precise iudgement.

⁋ The Summe of this boke.

The preface.
ordre of this boke.
How vrine is engendred in man, and how it passeth furth.
L.iij.

Of the Diuisiō and
Cap.i.
Chap.ij.
What

THE TABLE.

What vrine is and what tokens it geueth in generall   Chap. iij.
Of the forme of the vrinall, & of place
and tyme meete to iudge vrine, and
how it shulde be recepued.   Cap. iiij.
How menny thynges are to be considered in vrine.   Chap. v.
What a parfecte vrin is, and also how
menny wayes all partes of the
vrine may be altered in a helthfull
man.   Chap. vj.
What be the generall qualyties that
alter the partes of vrine.   Chap. vij.
Of the particuler causes of varietie in
euery vrine.   Chap. viij.
Of disforme Contentes.   Chap. ix.
Of the garlande & otherlyke thynges.
    the. x. Chapiter.
Of the commodities and medicines of
vrine.   the .xj. Chapiter.
Of the diseases touchynge vrine, & the
remedies of the same.   Chap. xij.
The composition & mixture of colours
how they are made.   Chap. xiij.
The declaration of certayn darke wordes apptaining to the arte of Physicke, vsed in this boke.   Chap. xiiij.

FINIS.

ℭ Imprinted at London in
Poules churche yarde,
at the sygne of the
Brasen Serpent
by Reynolde
Wolfe.

M. D. XLVII.

*Cum priuilegio ad imprimen=
dum solum.*

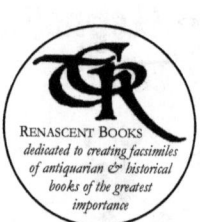

www.ingramcontent.com/pod-product-compliance
Lightning Source LLC
Chambersburg PA
CBHW061507180526
45171CB00001B/76